ACHIEVING UNLIMITED HEALTH

The baby boomers survival guide
in the new millennium?

Dr James Peter Cima

ISBN: 0692327126
ISBN 13: 9780692327128
Library of Congress Control Number: TXu942-946
Palm Beach Gardens, Florida

The Dedication

If you don't take care of your body,
where else are you going to live?

This book is dedicated to:

- ❖ My son, James, who said: "Dad, you have to let people know what you know...it would be a crime not to."
- ❖ My daughter, Natalie, who was so inspired by my work that she, too, became a doctor to carry on and further our research.
- ❖ All of my patients, their families, and their friends who have had to live or die through this difficult time.
- ❖ All the doctors who truly want to make a change in the health of this country.
- ❖ All the people who are sick and tired of being sick and tired.

If you don't take the time to take care of your
health, you will have to take the time to take care
of your sickness and disease!

Contents

The Foreword

Typically, for most of us, we enter this world in fairly good shape and have excellent health. There are those who are not as fortunate and are not as blessed but for the most part, when we are born, our bodies are functioning at a very high level of health.

We usually go through our childhood and our teenage years with minor health problems. When we hit our twenties and thirties, however, we continue to experience and encounter additional health problems, and any childhood problems continue to worsen. Around the fourth and fifth decades of life, our bodies start to break down rapidly. Any childhood or additional health problems that we encountered in our twenties or thirties may now become life threatening. This sets the stage for a very grave prognosis. This is the case with cancer and heart disease—two leading killers in our society today. These health problems are prevalent in many people, and those who are affected are dying from these diseases as early as thirty, forty, and fifty years old. When we hit our sixth and seventh decades, the many degenerative changes that have already riddled our bodies accelerate, and the downward spiral of life becomes a living nightmare.

Some of my patients tell me that their "golden years" are not so golden, and life is a "living hell on earth" for them. Their bodies and minds are so deteriorated and degenerated that death seems like the only way out. There are some people who may say we are living longer. This is debatable...and what is the quality of life at this point?

This is the reality of life as we experience it today. But is this really the reality, or is there another alternative? With the baby boomers approaching their fifth and sixth decades, they are looking for a new reality. They have watched their parents go down the road I described earlier, and they do not want to travel that same path. They are looking for a new reality. But unfortunately, you cannot have a new reality without a new plan; and you cannot have a new plan without a new vision. In other words, unless we change the way we view our health and how to condition our bodies to be healthy, we are all headed down that same dead-end road.

I don't think our creator wanted it this way. I don't think that life should end at sixty, seventy, or eighty when our bodies and minds have the capability to live much longer. Did you know that scientists say that the human body can live for at least 150–200 years? There are cells in your body that don't age, even though you may be eighty years old! In fact, the physiology textbook that is used in most medical schools suggests this:

Each of the 100 trillion cells in the human being is a living structure that can survive indefinitely and in most instances can even reproduce itself, provided its surrounding fluids simply remain constant.
—Arthur C. Guyton, MD
Guyton's Textbook of Medical Physiology

Your cells have the capability of living indefinitely. How long is indefinitely? I will let you determine that. But if this is the case, why are we dying so young? Hopefully this book will help you create that vision and outline a plan so that you, too, can live between 150 and 200 years, enjoying not only the quantity but also the quality of life. Before we do this, let's imagine what it would be like to live that long...

Imagine...

❖ Retiring at eighty and then spending the next 70–120 years retired.
❖ Playing your favorite sport at the age of one hundred and playing it better than you did when you were twenty.
❖ The wisdom that you would have at one hundred, so that the next fifty to one hundred years would be better lived than the first hundred.
❖ Playing with your great-great-great-great-grand-children.
❖ How many more things you could accomplish in and with your life if you doubled your life span.

❖ The technological advances that you could see in a lifetime.
❖ How wealthy you would be and how much fun you could have because you are healthy.

Imagine this new vision and a new dimension to your life!

Overview

Top Three Leading Causes of Death in the United States

1. Heart disease. According to the American Heart Association, cardiovascular disease claimed nine hundred and forty nine thousand six hundred and nineteen (949,619) lives in the United States in 1998. This is about a death a minute and takes more lives than the next seven causes of death combined. Things are getting worse, according to the American Heart Association in 2010 36.9% of the population have some form of cardiovascular disease and this will increase to 40.5% by 2030.
2. Cancer. According to the American Cancer Society, In 2013 Five hundred and eighty thousand three hundred and fifty (580,350) lives will be lost to cancer.
3. Iatrogenic diseases (physician induced), from the Greek term aɪˌætroʊˈdʒɛnɪk, which means "brought forth by the healer." Accounts for two hundred and fifty thousand lives per year according to the

Journal of the American Medical Association. When our treatment procedures are as dangerous or more so then the ailment you are being treated for, then you must think twice.

In order to see this new vision, let us first look at where we are. We have a health crisis on our hands. It's not because we need better health insurance or that there are too many people without health insurance. It's because we have to change the way we think and take care of our health, our most valued possession. The following are tough and sobering statistics to swallow:

❖ Approximately 4,800 people die each day from these three killers. Let me ask you a question, If accidental plane crashes claimed the lives of four thousand eight hundred Americans (4,800) per day would you fly?

❖ In one year, we lose approximately 1,751,819 Americans to these three killers.

Over fifty-six years of war we lost 1,648,248 Americans. In one year, we lose 103,571 more Americans to these killers than we lost in fifty-six years of war.

Total American War Casualties		
Revolutionary War	50,000	1775–1783 (eight years)
Civil War	970,000	1861–1865 (four years)
WWI	116,516	1914–1918 (four years)
WWII	405,399	1941–1945 (four years)
Pearl Harbor	2,390	1941 (one day)
Korean War	36,934	1950–1953 (three years)
Vietnam War	58,167	1959–1975 (sixteen years)
911	2,998	2001 (one day)
Iraq War	3,500	2003–2007 (four years)
Afghanistan	2,344	2001-2014 (thirteen years, counting)
Total	1,648,248	

Now, I realize that we cannot save everyone, but if we can prevent even 25 percent of the people in the prime of their lives from dying due to the above, then we will have saved 430,000 lives alone each year. So who do you think we should wage war against? Other countries? Or the three leading killers in our society today?

The choice is yours!

Section One:

Why Do We Rank So Low?

According to the World Health Organization, we rank thirty-seventh among nations in overall health and rank first in total cost per capita at $8,508 per person. So we are paying more for health care than any other nation, and we rank thirty-seventh among nations in overall health. Talk about being sick—thinking that the system we have now works is even sicker.

So, why do we rank so low in overall health? The simple truth is that doctors do not treat health; they treat sickness and disease. Long before modern medicine, when people became ill the focus was to get them well. Today, our focus is on curing the disease and not the patient. That statement may confuse you, but this is where the real *why?* begins. We took our focus off the cause and prevention of disease and focused on the disease instead. Doctors try to kill the disease instead of allowing the patient's body to overcome the disease. They try to medicate it out, burn it out, cut it out, or just plain beat it out of our bodies.

There is no principle of sickness and disease, only one of health. Let's stop pretending that there is a science of sickness and disease and realize that the only true science is health. The purpose of this book is encapsulated in that paradigm shift.

So, to reiterate, why do we rank so low in over-all health? The simple truth is that doctors do not treat health; they treat sickness and disease. Let me trace the anatomy of sickness and disease, which will include the scale of health and how doctors are trained to take care of health. I will then explain the new diagnostic methods and treatment plans that need to take place in order for our nation to achieve a higher level of health, our most valued possession.

I

The Anatomy of Sickness and Disease

B efore we can create a new vision for the health and wellness in this country, let's look at why this should be done. We will start from the beginning by first examining why and when someone would go to a doctor in the first place. Most people go to their doctor when they develop signs and symptoms. They do not realize that the unwanted health condition may have been there for years or decades before these signs and symptoms first appeared. This is a big part of why we rank thirty-seventh among nations in overall health. We were trained to wait for a symptom before going to the doctor. After all, this is how we were raised and trained by our society. We don't go to the doctor unless we have a problem known as a symptom. Even if you do go for your yearly checkup, it may not help based on what you will soon find out. Remember the statement below and brand it into your brain:

{ *Symptoms are the end result of a disease process, not the beginning.* }

If you do not get anything else out of this book, please remember the above statement! What most people fail to realize is that symptoms usually take years or even decades to develop. Waiting for symptoms to appear before a visit to your doctor is not a good idea if you want to maintain excellent health.

Do you know that ancient Asians paid their doctors to keep them well and didn't pay when they became sick? This is exactly opposite of what we do in the United States. We only pay our doctors when we get sick and never visit them when we are healthy, except for the occasional yearly physical. However, the yearly physicals are geared toward sickness and disease symptoms, not prevention. If you saw your doctor for your annual checkup and you had no symptoms, he or she would not know what to do with you. If you really wanted to puzzle your doctor, ask him or her what you could do to maintain excellent health. The unfortunate truth is that most doctors are trained in sickness and disease and not in obtaining excellent health. Remember, there is no principle of sickness and disease, only one of health.

On the next page is the scale of health that I developed many years ago. It shows you the stages of disease and how long it may take before symptoms appear. It is a realistic view of how we go from vibrant health to sickness, disease, and then death.

2

The Scale of Health

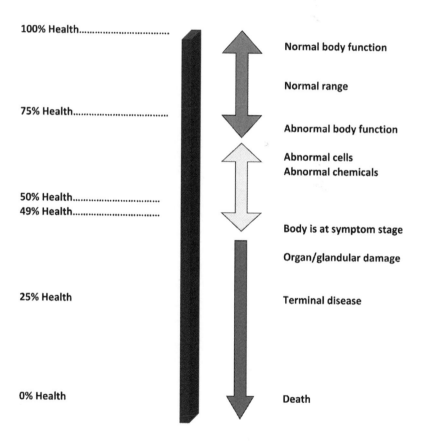

100% Health..................................   Normal body function

Normal range

75% Health..................................   Abnormal body function

Abnormal cells
Abnormal chemicals

50% Health..............................
49% Health..............................

Body is at symptom stage

Organ/glandular damage

25% Health   Terminal disease

0% Health   Death

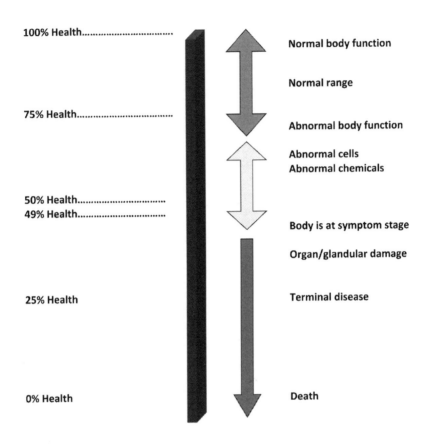

As you can see, the scale ranges from zero to one hundred, with zero being death and one hundred being peak performance and 100 percent health. The quality and quantity of your life depends on where you spend the majority of your time on this scale. If it is spent at a low percentage, then you will have many health problems, which will affect your life and hasten death. If it is spent at a high level, then your potential for survival is high, and you will live for a long time. Below are brief explanations of what each range represents:

100–75 Percent: The Functional Range

This is the range you should begin with at birth. The body is maintaining homeostasis (balance) and is doing well and succeeding. You have a lot of energy (both physically and mentally); you are happy and excited about life; and you are free of any pain or symptoms. Your body functions well; you are resilient; and you bounce back well from minor health problems. As stated above, most children begin here and stay here until their twenties.

75–50 Percent: Body Malfunction, Chemical, and Cellular Damage

In this range, the body is trying to cope with the stresses of life, which are physical, mental, and chemical. These stresses will be discussed in more detail, since they are the true causes of disease. Most people between the ages of twenty and forty are here. You feel OK; you know something is wrong; but you do not know what. At this point, your body has difficulty maintaining homeostasis (balance). The body starts to malfunction as your energy levels plummet. You may not have much to complain about except that you notice you may be aging prematurely. Your body is losing its shape, and you cannot eat the things or do the things you once did. Life loses meaning, and, to say the least, you are not a happy camper. Your overall state of well-being is down. A large percentage of our population falls into this category, which the medical profession has neglected.

50–25 Percent: Beginning of Symptoms and Life-Threatening Diseases

At this point in your health, your cells are undergoing damage at a rapid rate. Life-sustaining chemicals, such as hormones, enzymes, and antibodies, are altered, depleted, or absent. If the body is allowed to decline to 50 percent, this damage then leads to a state called disease. At 49 percent, the body desperately needs help, so it creates indicators in the form of symptoms. These symptoms can come in the form of chronic pain, headaches, fatigue, digestive disturbances, difficulty sleeping, or allergic reactions. If these symptoms are allowed to continue, the degeneration becomes worse, and the damage increases. As you inch your way down to 25 percent, you are classified as terminal, and the prognosis is dubious. At 25 percent and below, your body and mind begin to shut down. Eventually, you die when you reach 0 percent. These stages or levels start in your thirties, forties, and fifties and reach terminal levels in your forties, fifties, sixties, and seventies.

As you can see, symptoms occur way down the line. So, to make it simple:

1. It may take months to years for your body to start malfunctioning.
2. Malfunction leads to chemical changes taking place in your body over months or years.
3. Chemical changes lead to cellular damage over months or years.

4. Cellular damage eventually leads to symptoms, which will appear years or decades after the malfunctioning first occurred.

If you still don't believe that symptoms are the end result of a disease process, try this on for size. Try to buy life insurance after suffering from cancer or heart disease. Insurance companies will not sell life insurance to you. Do you know why? It's because you are considered a high risk. Even they know that symptoms are the end result.

Do you still need proof? Do you know what the first symptom of a heart problem is 30 percent of the time? It's *death!* Waiting for that impending heart attack is not the answer, because it does not give you time to react.

Still not convinced? Cancer is the second leading cause of death. It usually appears as a small lump (which takes from years to decades to develop), or you develop minor symptoms like abdominal discomfort or general fatigue. You go to the doctor, and he or she runs some preliminary tests just to see something that he or she "didn't like." The doctor sends you to a specialist, who runs more tests. Your worst nightmare becomes a reality as you learn from the doctor, weeks later, that you have a few months to live.

Waiting for symptoms to develop is not the answer. So what needs to be changed in order for us to improve the health of our society?

3

Using New Diagnostic Methods

The first problem we must conquer is developing diagnostic methods that diagnose a potential health problem before it becomes life threatening. Many of our diagnostic tools today do not detect health problems early enough. For example, an EKG does not diagnose an impending heart attack—it diagnoses the fact that you had a heart attack. A lot of good that's going to do after you're dead! An MRI diagnoses a bulging/herniated disc; it doesn't diagnosis a disc that has the potential to become herniated. A CT scan can find a tumor in the brain; however, it doesn't diagnose the possibility of a tumor developing. When your blood pressure is checked, it tells you that you already have high blood pressure, but it does not tell you why. Even our blood tests have reference ranges that are so broad that by the time you are out of the range, you have likely had a problem for many years.

So, most of our cutting-edge diagnostic methods give us information after we develop the disease and give us very little information about what to do to prevent the health condition from occurring in the first place. We must be able to diagnose and develop diagnostic tools that determine body malfunctions before chemical alterations

and cellular damage, when the body can still do something about what is happening. This will give us plenty of
time to do what is needed to be done. When waiting for
symptoms, we are just about out of time for the body to
retaliate and win over what is ailing it. So, changing our diagnostic methods will be necessary to create a new vision.

4

Changing Our Treatment Procedures and Protocols

The second change we must make is to change our treatment procedures and protocols. In order to understand this, let us go through a typical visit to the doctor's office.

Usually, the first thing you will do when a symptom or problem occurs is to try to diagnose yourself. You will either self-medicate or use some natural remedy that you've heard about through an article or a friend. Today, it's even worse, because you can use the Internet to learn more about your self-diagnosed condition, which adds even more to the confusion. Then, when you have had enough pain and suffering, you make an appointment to see your doctor. Finally, the day arrives, and you go to your doctor and fill out your paperwork. Your appointment is at 9:00 a.m., but you finally get to see the doctor at noon…if you are lucky. Usually, the doctor is pressed for time, underpaid and overworked, and he or she can only give you three minutes of her/his time. The doctor then has a nurse or physician's assistant give you a preliminary examination and may prescribe some tests (X-rays/MRI/CT scan, blood tests, EKG, etc.).

This whole process, from scheduling your appointment to getting all of your examinations and tests, may take from a few days to a few weeks. Finally, the doctor reviews all of your information and then comes up with a diagnosis. He or she then schedules you to come in for your consultation. At the consultation, the doctor reviews your findings, and he or she might as well be speaking in a foreign language, because you can only comprehend 20–30 percent of what the doctor is saying. The one thing that you do remember is your diagnosis. The *Merriam-Webster Dictionary* defines diagnosis as: "The art or act of identifying a disease from its signs and symptoms." For example, your doctor may say you have a diagnosis of a herniated disc, asthma, high blood pressure, migraine headaches, ulcers, etc. Please remember that a diagnosis does not tell you what caused your condition; it only labels your condition.

After the doctor diagnoses your symptoms, he or she will give you a medication that should improve your symptoms. If the medication does not work and doesn't cause other symptoms to occur or kill you, the doctor may give you a second, third, or fourth medication. This is usually done over the phone, without speaking to the doctor directly. At this point, you are spending more time with the pharmacist than the doctor. The cost of some of the medication is more than you make in a week, but you give them your credit card anyway.

When all these medications don't work, the doctor may send you out for more tests or send you to a specialist. Do you know what the definition of a specialist is? A doctor who knows more and more about less and less. By this time you may already have died or wished you had. Finally, the day of your appointment with the specialist arrives. You still have to fill out more forms, even though you bring a file cabinet with you containing your entire medical history and reports. The specialist will also take a case history, perform more exams, and run more tests. He/she will diagnose you again and either prescribe more medication or prescribe surgery. If surgery is prescribed, most people want a second opinion, and the whole cycle begins again. I could probably bore you with another three pages of this medical maze of health (sickness) care, but I think you get the picture.

Anyone who has ever been put through this maze would say that this is what typically happens. This is how our medical system works and has been working since the beginning. This is the model that we have all been embracing, and it appears to be the way that we should be treated. Now for the reality, the cold hard truth, where the rubber meets the road: it's what you do not see in what I have written above that may kill you. I am going to come up with some interesting points along the way, and you can either agree or disagree, based on what I bring up. You can decide on how you or a loved one would like to be treated.

Point 1: Symptoms

You are already behind the eight ball, because you are going to the doctor, and you already have symptoms. Remember, symptoms are the end result of a disease process, not the beginning. Unfortunately, you should have been there months, years, or decades prior, so that the doctor could have determined what was causing your problem. Then you would not be suffering from possible life-altering symptoms now. Like I stated before, ancient Asian doctors were paid to keep you well! Interesting concept, isn't it? This is much different from our medical model of health/sickness care today. In fact, it is much more cost-effective to treat people's health instead of their sickness and disease. Do you hear that Medicare, health insurance companies, and politicians? Maybe our premiums would become less if we followed the ancient Asian method of health care, but that might make some insurance companies and politicians angry.

Point 2: Examination and Testing

Doctors run more tests than ever before. These tests are extremely costly and usually don't determine the cause of the problem. Many patients that I see have negative test results but still have symptoms. This means that the testing procedures are not detailed enough to pick up malfunction or the beginnings of chemical or cellular damage. Oh, sure! They can see tumors, broken bones, heart damage, and gross pathology (damaged diseased tissues, glands, and organs), but they lack the ability to monitor body malfunction. What the medical establishment does not understand is that most of the testing that we do today, although technologically advanced and sophisticated, are not very successful at assessing a problem in the early stages of malfunction. In fact, there are many patients who go in for a physical and are given a clean bill of health but then drop dead of a heart attack as they are leaving the doctor's office.

So, although we have sophisticated equipment, tests and scans do not catch people in the malfunction state. At best, you have to be far down the trail leading to death before these tests are positive. We need examination tools that can determine health problems in the malfunctioning state. Einstein stated: *It takes a smart man to solve a problem, and it takes a brilliant man to prevent one.*

I feel that doctors should want to be brilliant so that they can prevent health problems.

Point 3: Diagnosis

Once the doctor comes up with a diagnosis, he or she brands you for life. Your diagnosis is with you until the day you die. I urge all of you to ask your doctors this question: "I am glad that you labeled my disease, and now it is part of me like a tattoo, but please tell me what is causing my label. How do we correct the cause so my body can cure itself?" The doctor will stand there flabbergasted, because he or she will not be able to answer your question with any kind of logic. The sad part isn't that they do not know the answer—it's that they don't want to know the answer, because it doesn't fit into their treatment regimen and the medical model.

I am sure I know what your doctor will say when you ask what is causing your diabetes, high blood pressure, or herniated disc, and what you can do to allow your body to heal itself and correct the cause of the problem. He/she will blame it on genetics, pollen, being overweight, your age, your work, or other reasons. He/she may say, "Stop this," or "Do that," but then will go no further. Doctors will not tell you specifically how to change your diet to help the body balance its biochemistry, and they certainly won't explain how and what types of exercise you should do. The truth is that they do not know, since they were never trained to do this. They will not explain to you how the body functions and what the body needs to be healthy, because they only know about sickness and disease and the use of drugs to treat the disease. When you talk health to most doctors, you might as well talk to them in another language. It is foreign to them to even think that way. They cannot even contemplate or understand what you are saying. This will annoy them, because they are the experts, and you are just the patient.

Just remember this…it's *your* body; it's *your* life, and it's *your* health. Never let anyone play games with your body, your health, and your life. Get the facts, and find a doctor who will intelligently answer your questions without getting angry or frustrated.

Point 4: Treatments: Drugs and Surgery

We will first look at drugs as a form of treatment and then surgery. Now, I want you to know that there are times when both of these treatments are necessary and can save your life. However, these should be used as a last resort when taking care of your health.

Drugs

Once you have a diagnosis, you are usually prescribed a drug. I want to make myself perfectly clear: I am not an advocate of drugs. In fact, I deplore them, and if I could take at least 50 percent of them off the market, I would! Let me clean this up and say that I am not against the use of drugs in some instances, but I am against the abuse of drugs in all instances. I agree there is a small (and I do mean small) portion of the population that may require drugs. Drugs should only be used when all natural alternatives are explored, and you should be taken off them as soon as possible. My personal opinion is that drugs are being abused by doctors as well as patients. But, the real culprits are the pharmaceutical firms. The pharmaceutical firms run the medical profession. Whatever the pharmaceutical firms say is gospel until they find out that a particular drug (which was the wonder drug of yesterday) is really a killer in our society. The drug is then pulled off the market ASAP only to be replaced by a new wonder drug, which will be taken off the market tomorrow. So, why are drugs so bad?

Drugs mask or hide symptoms. The interesting thing about medical treatment is that doctors give you a drug that will mask a symptom. You have high blood pressure; they give you something to lower it. You have low blood pressure; they give you something to elevate it. You have diarrhea; they give you something to constipate you. You are constipated; they give you something to cause diarrhea. Your sinuses are draining; they give you a drug to clog them. Your sinuses are clogged; they give you something to unclog them. You run a temperature; they have a drug that lowers it. That is how allopathic medicine (MDs) treat disease.

Why is this bad? Before I answer that question, let me ask you one. If your engine light came on and your car started to backfire, sputter, and spit out clouds of black smoke, would you immediately pull into a gas station to find out what is happening to your car? Now, if the mechanic checked your car and removed the fuse to the engine light so that the light went off, and he said, "OK, you're good to go," what would you say? Did he solve the problem? Or, did he just mask or hide the problem by removing the fuse so the engine light wouldn't go on? The obvious answer is that he did not find the problem but masked it by preventing the engine warning light from working. Had he taken the time to find out what was causing the engine problem and then corrected it, the light would not turn on, and your car would run fine.

This is what your doctor does when you present yourself at his office with a symptom. Doctors first label your condition and then give you a medication to mask it. They hide (mask) the symptom, giving you a false sense of security. You think you are fine, because your symptom is no longer apparent; however, your doctor never got to the cause of the symptom in the first place. Beside the fact that symptoms are the end result of a disease process, doctors mask it, allowing your condition to become more life-threatening. Does that make sense to you?

Most doctors do not realize the purpose of a symptom to begin with. The purpose of a symptom is a warning sign, just like the warning lights in your car. It means that the intelligence that runs your body is warning you that things are going badly, and the body is unable to deal with the cause. Your body creates a warning in the form of symptoms, letting you know the severity of what is going on. What a doctor must do is find out what is causing the symptom. Once you find and treat the cause, the symptom goes away and does not have to be hidden by a drug. Unfortunately, if doctors did this, the drug companies would literally go out of business. It would be a shame for them, but the health of our nation would improve.

Drugs interfere with the normal function of the body. People do not realize that the drugs they take interfere with bodily functions. The human body is a true masterpiece of function. It is composed of one hundred trillion cells that are controlled by fifty billion brain cells through an interconnecting system of nerves in which the possible number of nerve pathways is the number one followed by fifteen thousand zeroes. With pinpoint accuracy, these cells carry on all the functions that occur in your body constantly. It has been said that if you had a hard copy of all bodily functions over a twenty-four-hour period, it would cover the surface of the earth. Can you imagine interfering with that type of function?

Did you know that your body has its own pharmaceutical firm? Your body produces all the chemicals that it needs for survival. In fact, all pharmaceutical drugs are knockoffs of chemicals that your body produces. Your body produces hormones, pain suppressants, mood elevators, its own form of antibiotics, blood pressure medications, and digestive aids, to name a few. My question would be: Why isn't my body producing the chemicals that it should be producing? Before I would put a chemical into my body, I would want to know the answer to that question. Once that question is answered, I would want to know the answer to my next question: What can be done to get my body to produce that chemical?

So let's look at a group of medications called synthetic hormones and see how they interfere with body function. These synthetic hormones are used to treat many conditions, such as diabetes (insulin), thyroid gland weakness (synthroid), male sterility (testosterone), female problems (estrogen and progesterone), and stunted growth (growth hormone). Isn't it funny that doctors can prescribe the same hormones that your body produces? Why is this not a good thing?

First of all, the hormones are usually synthetic (fakes), and from a chemical perspective, they do not function like the real thing. It would be like trying to put a left-handed glove on your right hand. It will fit but will not let your hand function very well. Synthetic hormones will chemically function in your body but not as effectively as the real thing.

Secondly, because you are giving your body hormones, those glands producing the hormones will literally atrophy and become weaker. For example, if you exercise a muscle, it gets bigger and stronger. If you stop exercising that muscle, it shrinks. If you become totally sedentary, it will atrophy. The same holds true if we have a glandular problem. Let's say a woman's ovaries are not producing normal amounts of female hormones. By giving her the synthetic hormone, it will make her glands shut down even faster than if she had not been given the hormone.

Thirdly, hormones are time-released into the body. In other words, they are released throughout the day, sometimes at an increased rate and sometimes at a decreased rate. When you take a pill, you are releasing the entire hormone at one time. Why is this bad? Hormones act along with other hormones in what they call feedback mechanisms, where the increase of one hormone will decrease another hormone, and this hormone may increase another, and this will affect another and another—you get the picture. When you just put all the hormone in at once, you create a cascade of other hormonal imbalances in the body as well, creating other diseases.

My questions are: Why is this gland malfunctioning? What can I do to heal the gland? Once you find the cause, then you can correct it, and the gland will be able to produce its own hormones, and the symptoms will disappear.

Not only do drugs mask your symptoms and interfere with normal body function, but they also cause side effects (diseases) as well, leading to even more symptoms (some of which are worse than the symptoms you were suffering from to begin with). Some side effects are so bad that death can be the result! I don't know about you, but if the treatment is worse than the disease, then I don't want it. For example, some well-known drugs can cause heart attacks, strokes, cancer, liver disease, kidney problems, and neurological degeneration. Every symptom that you manifest because of a drug is causing potential damage to other organs, glands, systems, and body parts. As if this were not bad enough, most doctors have no idea about the potential side effects of drug interactions. For example, they may know that drug A can cause certain diseases and that drug B can cause some other diseases. However, when these two drugs interact, they may create a new set of diseases that may be different from those created by drugs A and B alone. Doctors have no way to know what will happen or how you will respond when you take drugs. How is that for the scientific treatment of your condition?

You may take the drug and have your symptoms reduced; the drug may do nothing; or, you may die, go into anaphylactic shock, or suffer a heart attack. Neither you nor your doctor will know the outcome until after the fact. Is that how you want to be treated?

Meanwhile, if you take a drug and develop another symptom or disease, your doctor is more than willing to give you another drug to mask the new symptom or disease that you just developed from the first drug you were taking. The new drug also has side effects, which will create new symptoms. It's like the dog chasing its tail; it is a never-ending cycle. One day you will be on more drugs than your body can take, eventually leading to death.

Surgery

I always found it hard to accept that a patient would benefit from the removal of organs, glands, discs, and joints. Again please let me reiterate I am not against the use of surgeries, but I am against the abuse of surgeries. Being knocked unconscious, sliced open, and having part of your body removed for no logical reason sounds more like a nightmare than a treatment procedure. The reality is this is what is happening to millions of Americans in hospitals every year. People are having organs and body parts removed like it is no big thing and sometimes without reason, and for what? Why are we so willing to submit our bodies to a doctor wielding a very sharp knife? Because the doctor thought it was the right thing to do? We should show a little more concern and restraint when it comes to surgery. It's OK for you to be skeptical and to want all the information you can get before making that decision. The bottom line: surgery is not something to be taken lightly. When confronted with the option of surgery, it's important for you to remember that you have a choice. Don't just trust the opinion of one doctor; get a second and third opinion. It could mean the difference between life and death.

Once a surgical procedure is performed, in most cases, your body will never function as well without that organ, gland, or joint. For example, once a gland such as your thyroid, ovaries, uterus, tonsils, appendix, kidney etc. is removed, no matter how much you try, your health will never be the same. Let's face it: God, in his or her infinite wisdom, gave each of us these organs, glands, and joints for proper body function. Once they are removed, at best, your health becomes a crap shoot. What this means is that you and your doctor cannot fully predict the implications of this surgery. Once that organ or gland is removed, it will have far-reaching effects on many other body parts and functions, which will lead to many disease processes that could have been prevented if that organ had been saved. Now I know what some of you might be thinking, especially if you've gone under the knife. You might say that my joint, organ, and gland was so diseased or damaged and I had so much pain and suffering that it had to come out. I would agree to a certain extent, but if I were to ask you if that organ, gland, or joint could have been saved before it reached that dangerous point, would you have wanted to save that organ or gland? Or would you still have chosen surgery? If you are sane, the answer is obvious.

Remember, you run the risk of serious health consequences that may be worse than the unwanted health condition you now have. Accidents happen, and if you are the unfortunate one, then you may become a statistic. Many times after surgery, patients became paralyzed or otherwise mentally or physically handicapped due to a mistake during surgery. Doctors and nurses are human, too, and they sometimes make mistakes, which may cost you your health. The Harvard University School of Public Health estimates that as many as 1.3 million Americans suffer disabling injuries in hospitals yearly, and 198,000 of those may result in death. Seven out of ten of those deaths were preventable—48 percent from faulty surgery and a third from negligence.

You may be required to undergo additional surgeries. Many times I have seen patients that have had multiple back surgeries, and the sad truth is that these patients are still in pain. I have also seen patients that undergo multiple joint replacement surgeries, starting with the one hip, then the other hip, then one knee, etc. This usually occurs later on in life when, it becomes difficult to bounce back from surgery.

The cost of surgery and the road to recovery may have devastating financial consequences. Many patients do not have insurance and have to pay out of pocket, sometimes shelling out tens of thousands to hundreds of thousands of dollars. This can literally ruin you financially and create hardships on many family members.

You may die. The American College of Surgeons and the American Surgical Association suggested that 30 percent of operations performed each year were unnecessary; 50 percent of the remaining procedures were beneficial but not essential to save or extend the patient's life. In all, it was thought that the needless and dubious operations were causing an unnecessary thirty thousand deaths per year. The unnecessary expenses and deaths become noticeable when doctors are in short supply or go on strike. In such cases, the death rate in an area can drop remarkably, much to the embarrassment of the medical community (when the facts can't be covered up).

Surgery does not get to the cause of the health problem. The sad reality is that the cause for the surgery is never determined. For example, your doctor may have told you that you need a hysterectomy, but he or she never told how the uterus became diseased in the first place. The same goes for your gall bladder, appendix, spinal condition, etc. So whatever caused your diseased organ remains in your body even though the organ was removed. This cause, left unchecked, can now manifest or disguise itself as something entirely different and will rear its ugly head in the future with life-threatening consequences. I have encountered many patients who, after their surgical procedures, develop more serious health problems later on in life, requiring additional surgeries.

5

The Choice Is Yours!

Hopefully you now have a better idea of the question that I asked at the beginning of this section, which is: Why do we rank so low among nations and countries in our overall health? The simple truth is that doctors do not treat health; they treat sickness and disease. That is where the *why* begins. So how do we reverse this already diseased and perverted health care cycle?

Demand a right of choice.

We should have a right to choose what type of care we want. At this point, you have very little choice, if any. You are pigeonholed into believing that the medical route is the only way to go. Over the past thirty-five years, I have seen a lot of people whose lives have been cut short and the quality decreased to a living nightmare. I am so appalled by this treachery and cannot believe it is happening here in the United States. Doctors are so numb and brainwashed that they really believe that their way is the only way. The general public is so accustomed to believing in their doctors and the medical system that they readily follow recommendations that can destroy the quality and quantity of their lives. They will even go as far as praising their procedures, treatments, and doctors for destroying their lives. The most amazing thing to me is when patients who are on their deathbeds rave about their care, even though the treatment caused their demise.

It is our God-given right to free speech and a right to demand a choice in health care. Just like we have a two-party system in our government, we must demand a two-party system in our health care. Just imagine if we only had Democrats or Republicans running the country. It would not be the democracy that we now live in. It would be one-sided and would cause our country to be unstable, weak, and prone to fail. The fact that we have this two-party system keeps the country balanced, and since each part has an equal footing with the other, it helps to maintain this balance. So, we must demand this change in our society for the betterment of our health care system.

The remainder of this book is an educational tool for the patient or layperson to use in understanding what health is and what you can do to help improve your health and that of your families. I hope you will be as excited and energized when you read this book as I was when I wrote it. I also hope that you can feel my message and the overwhelming enthusiasm I felt when I was writing it for you. Here's to a long successful journey to optimal health!

Wishing you the best of health,
Dr. James P. Cima

The Reason

The Reason Why I Wrote This Book

Being involved in the health field for over thirty-seven years has been an eye-opening experience for me. When I first entered practice in 1977, the United States ranked seventeenth among nations in overall health. I asked myself why. We have the best hospitals, the most highly trained and skilled doctors, and we spend millions of dollars on research. We have more knowledge in the health field than any ten nations put together. Why, with all that we know, do we rank so low?

Today, thirty-seven years later, we supposedly have even more knowledge, better hospitals, better drugs, spend billions and our doctors have a better education and even more skills than they had thirty-seven years ago. We have more sophisticated procedures and diagnostic equipment than we did thirty-seven years ago. So, why did we drop twenty places to be ranked thirty-seventh among nations in overall health? Why are we going in the wrong direction? The reasons will astound you! The *why* is my reason for writing this book.

To be truly educated means to have one's insight deepened and not to have one's information increased. It means to have a clearer and greater understanding, compassion, and empathy for the human race and their problems.
—L Ron Hubbard

Section Two:

Achieving Unlimited Health

Is It Possible to Achieve Unlimited Health and Double the Present Human Life Span?

I not only think that it is possible but that there are people alive today who will live for at least 150 years. I also believe that the quality of our years will increase along with the quantity.
—Dr. James P. Cima

Let us also focus on enjoying life as well—living every day like it is our last and planning for the future as though we were going to live forever.
—Dr. James P. Cima

Each of the 100 trillion cells in the human being is a living structure that can survive indefinitely and in most instances can even reproduce itself, provided its surrounding fluids simply remain constant.
—Arthur C. Guyton, MD
Guyton's Textbook of Medical Physiology

Learn the secrets of metabolic stimulation that can transform your body, mind, health, and life.
—Dr. James P. Cima

6

The Elusive Fountain of Youth

Is it possible to achieve unlimited health and double the present human life span? I believe so! I also believe that there are people alive today who will live for at least 150 years. I also believe that the quality of our years will improve along with the quantity. It is interesting to note that our present life span of approximately seventy-eight years has almost doubled what it was during the nineteenth century. At that time, the average life span was only forty-seven years. Life expectancy rose close to our present-day level back in the 1960s at approximately seventy years of age. Over the past fifty-four years, the average life span has increased very little despite great advances in modern-day medicine. Although we have made great strides since the beginning of the twentieth century, it appears that we have hit the proverbial brick wall. By the time most people reach their midfifties and sixties, their bodies have started to undergo life-threatening degenerative processes, such as cancer or heart disease. Even if we are fortunate to live past this mark, the quality of life sometimes leaves much to be desired. Our physical and mental capabilities diminish rapidly, accompanied by pain and a myriad of symptoms. To some, death may seem like the easy way out. To be honest, I do not think God intended for us to suffer like this during our so-called golden years. I say it is time for a change. At the beginning of the new millennium, why not think about doubling the average life span, just like we did one hundred years ago, and live to be 150.

Listen, we doubled the average life span in the nineteenth century. Why not double it again in the next century? This time, let us not only double our life span but improve the quality of our lives as well. Let us focus on our well-being so that our physical and mental capabilities mature like a fine wine, just hitting our stride at the hundred-year mark. Let us also focus on enjoying life as well—*living every day like it is our last and planning for the future as though we were going to live forever.* This should be our new motto. I am sure all of us, if we had the choice, would choose this type of lifestyle. The purpose of this book is not just to give you hope; I also want to demonstrate that your body and mind possess the capabilities of unlimited health.

7

The Purpose of Life

A ccording to Elbert Hubbard, life is "one damn thing after another." That is an interesting concept, but not the one I want to explore. The purpose of life is survival. The opposite of life is death. In order to prevent death, you must do things to improve your health in order to survive. There are a number of levels that one must survive on, but for our discussion, let us agree that the healthier you are, the greater your potential for survival is.

> *Each of the 100 trillion cells in the human being is a living structure that can survive indefinitely and in most cases can even reproduce itself, provided its surrounding fluids simply remain constant.*
> *—Arthur C. Guyton, MD*
> Guyton's Textbook of Medical Physiology

Most people want to live and would not mind living forever if it were possible. Therefore, there is a built-in mechanism in each of us that is always striving to survive. Everything you think, say, and do, to some degree, is based on how it will affect your survival. Right at this very moment, the body is trying to survive. Your body continually tries to right itself, regardless of the circumstances. In science, we call this "maintaining homeostasis." In other words, our body chemistry is always trying to accommodate (reorganize) and adjust to our environment. Our bodies maintain this state of homeostasis through a process known as metabolism.

Metabolism is the sum total of bodily processes that are necessary to maintain body function, thus maintaining life. Let me explain. Metabolism is a two-part process, and its two phases are known as anabolism and catabolism. Your body experiences wear and tear, just like anything else (cars, houses, and clothes), and it is always repairing itself from the stresses and strains of life. The only difference is that your body has the ability to tear down, repair, rebuild, and renovate itself every six months to a year. That's right! You have a brand-new body every six months to a year. You have a new heart, muscles, skin, bones, liver, stomach, etc. This is a normal part of life. Every day, cells are used up, and chemicals are broken down (catabolism), and every day new cells replace the old cells, and new chemicals are produced to replace the old chemicals (anabolism). You might now ask if this is the case and everything is so new, why do I look so old? I will answer that next.

The balance between catabolism and anabolism determines the speed at which you age. To avoid aging rapidly, your anabolic process must, at the very least, keep up with your catabolic process. If catabolism is greater than anabolism, you have a problem. The body is breaking down (aging) faster than the body is rebuilding itself, and this creates premature aging, sickness, disease, and death. However, if anabolism is greater than catabolism, you have maturity, health, growth, and repair. As mentioned above, anabolism is your building-up phase, and catabolism is your breaking-down phase. The process of anabolism includes replenishing energy, creating all chemicals necessary to sustain life, and repairing and rebuilding cells.

> *To improve your anabolic phase, you must have:*
>
> ❖ *Proper mental/emotional and physical stimulation*
> ❖ *Proper mental/emotional and physical rest*
> ❖ *Proper nutrition to repair and rebuild the body*

Ideally, the building-up process should be greater than the breaking-down process, especially when high demands are placed on the body. As you can see, if you manipulate metabolism, you can speed up or slow down the aging process.

Metabolic Manipulation

If I can show you how to slow catabolism by 50 percent and improve your anabolism by that same amount, you will increase your life span by 100 percent!

Did you get that? If I can show you how to slow catabolism by 50 percent, and improve your anabolism by that same amount, you will increase your life span by 100 percent! Metabolic manipulation is a term I coined to describe how to slow down the aging process. The elusive fountain of youth that Ponce de Leon went in search of was within us all along. This book will guide you through the steps of metabolic manipulation. It will help you learn to:

- ❖ Slow down catabolism or cannibalism (when your body feeds off itself, such as with cancer).
- ❖ Build up your anabolic phase and make it much more powerful than it is now.

If you follow the ideas and principles in this book, you will see a dramatic change in how you feel and look. With this in mind, we can at least establish the fact that the more we do toward survival, the better and longer that survival can be. Not only will our life span be lengthened but the quality and enjoyment will be overwhelming. Most of us want to live a long, healthy, and prosperous life. Our next step is to define what life is, since this is what we want to achieve.

8

The Triune of Life

The Essence of Life

Did you ever wonder about the differences between someone who is alive and someone who is dead? Or, for that matter, the difference between an inert substance, such as a rock, and a living being? More specifically, what are the necessary ingredients that compose life? These questions can be answered by the triune of life. A triune is defined as "consisting of three in one or a united group of three." A triune, then, is a group of three that creates a particular thing, and in this text, that thing is life. The three necessary ingredients or properties that life must possess are:

1. Infinite intelligence (spirit)
2. A physical body
3. A force or energy that bonds this infinite intelligence to the physical body

Let us touch on each side of this triune so you can get a better picture of what the essence of life is.

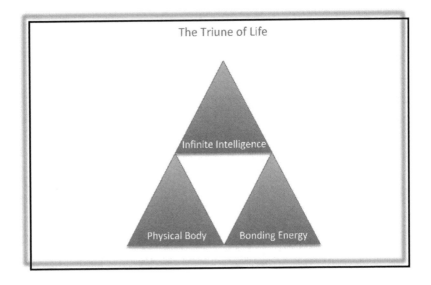

The First Essence of Life

Life Possesses Infinite Intelligence; Death Does Not.

This is rather obvious. A live human can think. A corpse cannot. More importantly, a living being is capable of organizing and reorganizing its body chemistry and repairing and rebuilding the physical body, by eating food. This allows the body to adapt to the environment around it. A corpse cannot do any of this and eventually decays. So, therefore, a living being possesses the power of thought and the inherent, or built-in, intelligence to organize and reorganize itself to perpetuate life. This intelligence therefore is the cause of thought and uses your brain as the organ to think, just like this intelligence uses your stomach to digest food you eat.

Life Requires a Physical Body, Capable of Function, Repair, and Rebuilding.

The Second Essence of Life

A corpse cannot perform any of the above. At this point, you realize that in order to have life, we must have intelligence. The purpose of that intelligence is to create in nine months a physical body from two simple cells; one called a sperm the other an ovum. The purpose of this physical body is to house this intelligence and to provide an operating base from which this intelligence can function in the physical universe. Our bodies, then, are necessary to support and house this intelligence. Conversely, our intelligence allows our bodies to replicate, perpetuate, and function in a way to support this intelligence, allowing life to continue. Your body is the *temple* of this intelligence, and this intelligence runs your body and your mind.

By the way, this intelligence has been given many different names, such as: the spirit, innate intelligence, thetan, elan vital, vital force, etc. Whichever name you use, just remember that these terms are interchangeable.

Life Must Possess a Biochemical Electrical Magnetic Force Field. This Is Where Life Meets Death.

The Third Essence of Life

The third essence of life deals with the bonding energy (force) that is noted and measured between the physical body and this infinite intelligence. Today, the legal medical definition of death is when there are no longer any brain impulses. This is verified by an instrument known as an EEG (electroencephalograph). An EEG measures your brain waves—the electrical energy that your brain produces. No energy, no brain waves, and you are pronounced dead, done, finito! So the one true legal distinction between life and death is this: When there is no biochemical, electrical magnetic energy in the brain to allow the body to function, you are dead. Experiments performed at Penn State University back this up. Researchers used the electrical energy from a rabbit's brain to run a radio. The radio worked until all of the electrical energy in the rabbit's brain was used up. When that happened, not only did the radio stop playing but the rabbit died. It also appears that anything that weakens this biochemical electrical bond may cause death or, if you are lucky, only sickness and disease.

So, life is a triune that is composed of an intelligence, a body, and this cohesive electrical energy. Remove any element and you, in an instant, go from life to death. For example, damage the physical body beyond repair, and the body cannot support this intelligence; death follows. Drain the electrical energy out of the body, and death ensues. Anything that would cause this infinite intelligence to be separated (severed) from the body leads to sickness, disease, and then death.

I hope this gives you a better understanding of the essence of life. Now that you understand what life is made of, let us discuss how you can improve the quality and quantity of your life. The healthier you are, the greater the quality and quantity of your life. In fact, there is no other indicator that can monitor your life better than your health. Health, then, becomes our next topic of interest and our next chapter.

9

Health: Your Most Valued Possession

{ *Your survival potential is proportionate to your health.* }

I s there anything more important than your health? If you answered no, you're on the right track. Let me make one thing perfectly clear: healthy people have a greater ability to survive or "live." Healthy people rarely get sick. Healthy people have more energy. Healthy people enjoy life. Healthy people are successful. Do you know why? They value their lives, and they know that without health, there is no life.

You should realize two important points before we continue. The first is that nothing is more valuable than your health. The second is that you know little or nothing about health and less about how to care for it. No offense intended, but these { *Healthy people do not die from sickness and disease; sick people do.* } are the facts. The purpose of this book is to address and explore these issues. The quantity and quality of your life are directly proportionate to your health. Therefore, it is paramount that your health be a primary focus in your life.

You have to devote time to studying and caring for your most valued possession. This is something you will enjoy doing, because you will feel better and look great. These are the same reasons that motivate you to do other things. You like to do things that make you feel and look good, don't you? By taking care of your health, you will feel great and will want to continue doing what makes you feel great.

As you read this book and learn the tools necessary to enhance your health, your health will improve. When you start to apply the principles at your own pace, you will see improvements in your health and life. Most people do not know how to take care of their health, because they were never taught how. In fact, their viewpoint on health is not one of wellness but of sickness and disease. People tend to confuse health, sickness, disease, and the body's capability in the healing process. I would like to address the following points in order to give you a more complete picture of health. I will:

1. Define health.
2. Examine the triune of health.
3. Teach you how to achieve unlimited health.

10

The Definition of Health

Health is a condition of wholeness in which the body functions at nearly 100 percent of its capacity chemically, physically, mentally, emotionally. Health is not merely the absence of symptoms.

When I ask people if they are healthy, most of the time they say yes. You probably think you are healthy. Whether you are or not makes no difference. This is how most people answer. If I feel good or OK, I am healthy. Alternatively, if I look or feel sick, then I am not healthy. A thorough physical exam may prove otherwise, but this is how people tend to think. Most people rely on how they feel, look, or a combination of both to assess their health. Why do you think this way? This is how you learned to monitor your health. Feelings can be misleading. The way you feel and look are indicators, but they have many limitations. Relying solely on them leaves you playing Russian roulette with your health and your life.

> *Feeling or looking good does not mean that you are healthy. And experiencing symptoms does not mean that you are sick.*

Just as I stated earlier, people have the erroneous idea that if you have no symptoms, you are healthy. Nothing could be farther from the truth. Although you probably grew up with this belief, please remove it from your mind, because it is not true. Replace it with this very important truth: symptoms are the end result of a disease process, not the beginning.

If you now have symptoms, let me give you some tips on what you should do.

Symptoms—Friend or Foe?

Most people do not like symptoms, because they are uncomfortable. But they do serve a purpose. Allow me to explain why you need to embrace symptoms rather than eliminate them, especially when you or your doctor has not identified what caused the symptom in the first place. When you develop a symptom, your body is warning you that you have a problem that you must deal with immediately, or more harm will come. The more discomfort, the greater the damage. It is your body's defense system at work. Something is causing your body to malfunction at an uncontrollable level, and you had better find the cause immediately. Can you imagine if we did not have this warning system in place? We would be an accident waiting to happen.

Now that you have the symptom and you realize its importance, try not to mask or hide it with medication or surgery, because the problem usually goes downhill from here. What you must do is find the cause of that symptom. Please note that the cause of the problem is not the symptom. The symptom is only the reflection of that cause and not the cause itself. Let me explain what I mean: If you have pain (a symptom), you must look for the cause of that pain before you start medicating the pain. If you experience a high temperature, you had better find out what is causing the body to react that way in the first place before you start to lower it.

Symptoms are similar to the indicator lights in your car. The oil light goes on, and you know that there is a malfunction. If you ignore that light, even for a little while, it could mean serious damage that requires a new engine or, in your body's case, a new hip, heart, etc. If you ignore symptoms, thinking that they are going to go away, guess what? They will stay, sometimes continually. Sometimes they even fool you and disappear only to rear their ugly heads later when they become life-threatening. Therefore, although symptoms are uncomfortable, they aid us in understanding that the body is not functioning properly. Then we can determine the cause. Time is the only problem with symptoms, since you do not have much of it. Remember: symptoms are the end result of a disease process, not the beginning. So, to experience excellent health and live to be 150, symptoms are not reliable indicators. Follow the tips above and get to the cause.

Now that I have outlined what health is not, let us now turn to what health is:

> Health:
> A condition of wholeness
> in which the body/mind
> functions at peak performance
> chemically, physically, and
> mentally emotionally as a
> triune in perfect harmony.

II

The Triune of Health

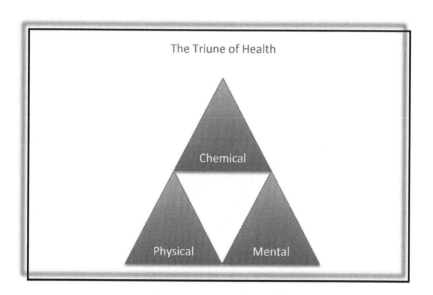

When you think health, I want you to think chemical, physical, and mental/emotional. In order for you to be healthy in body and mind, these factors have to be balanced. The converse is also true. In order for you to be sick, you must be out of balance chemically, physically, and mentally/emotionally. To become well again, you must use the proper chemical, physical, and mental components to restore that balance. Each human being is made up of a chemical entity (we are a cauldron of bio-chemical reactions), a physical entity (our body), and a mental entity (our mind). Our health is a composite: one-third chemical, one-third physical, and one-third mental. Therefore, if you eat well but you are stressed out, then you are not healthy mentally. If you exercise and eat like a pig, then you are not healthy chemically. If you eat great and do not exercise, you cannot be healthy physically. You must balance each entity if you want to have excellent health. Remember, every day your body and mind are being stressed (broken down) by chemical, physical, and mental/emotional factors. Therefore, you must stimulate or condition yourself chemically, physically, and mentally/emotionally every day if you want to be healthy. I will discuss this below in more detail. As long as you provide the necessary ingredients chemically, physically, and mentally/emotionally, your body will always strive to maintain health, since this is the essence of life.

Your body is constantly and persistently trying to maintain health, for health brings life and survival. In the scientific world, we call this homeostasis. As stated in the previous chapter, we all possess a magical power that heals the body. Religious groups call it the "spirit." Chiropractic physicians call it "innate intelligence." Others call it "elan vital," or vital force. The Egyptians called it "chu," the ancient Chinese called it "qi," and still others call it "chief prana." I do not care what you call it. Just realize that it does exist and is an ever-present power or "infinite wisdom" in the body that is constantly trying to maintain homeostasis in order to keep your body working properly.

What is interesting is that you, mentally and emotionally, are doing things right now, consciously and unconsciously, that are harming your body. Moreover, this magical power of perfection is always trying to defend your body against whatever harm has been done. For example: mentally, you may decide to drink alcohol, take drugs, or eat fast food. Now this supreme intelligence has the task of compensating for these problems to maintain some type of balance. You may have started coughing the first time you smoked. The coughing was this infinite wisdom telling you that the smoke was harmful to your body. Your mental intelligence told you to do this because your friends smoked. Sometimes your body can maintain balance, and sometimes it cannot. At a certain point, the body can no longer maintain balance chemically, physically, and mentally/emotionally. If the abuse is bad enough, you get sick or die.

We talk about spousal and child abuse. What about body abuse? If body abuse were a crime, 95 percent of the population would be doing time in jail. You know what the irony is? You are doing time; you just don't know it. Your spirit lives in a body that needs help desperately, especially if you are suffering from pain or a myriad of symptoms. Living in a body like this is doing time. Wouldn't you agree?

So not only does your body possess the power to heal itself, it has a built-in mechanism to maintain survival. Your body wants to survive. Now that you know that your body constantly tries to maintain itself regardless of how hard you try otherwise, you must now determine the following:

1. What would you have to do, chemically, physically, and mentally/emotionally to give your body what it needs to maintain health?
2. How can you continue to evaluate and reevaluate your progress for as long as you want to live, without relying on symptoms?

This is a way of life that demands your time, attention, and wisdom. You cannot, in all honesty, trust anyone with your health. You have been duped into believing that your body takes care of itself without your help and that when you have a problem, a doctor can heal you. You have to learn to listen to the doctor inside you, who heals you every day. This is what this book is about—giving the doctor inside what is needed to heal the body. Then find a doctor of the future to evaluate and reevaluate your health chemically, physically, and mentally/emotionally. Your doctor should then advise and apprise you of what you should do to create balance. Then, you should follow the advice and monitor your health, following the principles in this book, always listening to the intelligence that runs your body.

At this point, I would like to address the rest of the health triune and, more specifically, discuss the chemical, physical, and mental/emotional sides of this triune.

The Cause, Cure, and Treatment of All Disease

The cause of all malfunction, disease, and symptoms are chemical, physical, and mental/emotional stresses exerted on the body. Below is a list of chemical, physical, and mental/emotional stresses that cause disease.

Chemical Causes That Lead to Disease:

- ❖ Restricted calories or fad diets.
- ❖ Eating processed or chemically altered foods.
- ❖ Overeating.
- ❖ Alcohol and/or drugs (medical or street drugs).
- ❖ Smoking.
- ❖ Environmental pollutants found in our air, water, food, and clothes.

All of the above deplete, destroy, or remove the vital nutritional reserves of our bodies. This prevents our normally occurring chemical reactions from taking place, which leads to organ and glandular malfunction, disease, and symptoms.

Physical Causes That Lead to Disease:

- ❖ Falls/accidents/trauma
- ❖ Sports injuries
- ❖ Occupational hazards
- ❖ Excessive body weight
- ❖ Lack of exercise or too much or the wrong kind

The above are all considered physical causes due to the effects of gravity and the laws of physics. These stresses physically damage or displace muscle, tendon, nerve, ligament, gland, organ, or bone tissue, causing a variety of organ/glandular problems, body pains, aches, and stiffness. These conditions lead to organ and glandular degeneration (heart disease/cancer), joint degeneration, disc disease, and crippling arthritis.

Mental/Emotional Causes That Lead to Disease:

❖ Family
❖ Finances
❖ Friends
❖ Health problems
❖ Professional/work

Mental/emotional states, such as hostility, pain, anger, fear, grief, and apathy trigger nerve impulses that travel to organs and glands. For example, when you are angry, your heart will beat faster, and your blood pressure will elevate. If you are in a constant state of anger, this effect on your body could take years off your life. The same is true for people who are unhappy/depressed, etc. Their glands/organs slow down, leading to decreased hormonal/enzyme levels, then to body malfunction, sickness, and disease.

Choosing the Right Side

When you determine the cause or causes of your health problem, be sure to pick the right side of the tri-une. Look at the causes listed thus far, and determine which are the likely stresses or causes of your health problems. This will help you search for the right answers that lie within the pages of this book. Please note: if you choose the wrong cause, then you will pick the wrong treatment and will not get rid of your problem. You will know if you picked the wrong cause, because your health problem will usually remain. Therefore, pain caused by a physical fall needs physical treatment for a successful outcome. Pain medicine, although it will reduce the pain, will not remove the cause. The cause of all disease, from a hangnail to cancer, stems from chemical, physical, and/or mental/emotional stresses that can exert overwhelming damage to the body.

So:

❖ All disease is caused by any and all of the same three factors.
❖ All cures come from these three factors.
❖ All doctors, regardless of type, from a medical doctor to a witch doctor, treat you through the same three factors.

To give you a better illustration, let's examine how all doctors treat their patients. Regardless of the type of physician (medical, chiropractic, dental, naturopathic, acupuncturist), the treatment would be chemical, physical, or mental/emotional. You decide for yourself which treatment you want.

Chemical Cures and Treatment

For example, a medical doctor could treat you chemically with medications, such as painkillers, antibiotics, anti-inflammatory drugs, antidepressants, chemo, etc. All medications are "chemicals" that doctors use to treat chemical imbalances in the body. A doctor such as a chiropractic physician can also treat you chemically to enhance your health through proper diet and food supplementation, such as vitamins, minerals, herbs, homeopathic remedies, and tissue concentrates, which are used to help the body heal itself. The reason I like the use of nutrition to balance my body chemistry is obvious:

- ❖ Food gives my body the necessary raw materials for growth, repair, chemical production, and energy.
- ❖ Food supplements can help make up for deficiencies in my diet and help heal specific chemical imbalances.
- ❖ Food and food supplementation have little or no adverse reactions.
- ❖ You can work with a person nutritionally without waiting for the symptomatic stage.

These are the two methods of chemical care that physicians offer. You decide which care you want. If you want to live for 150 years, the answer is obvious.

Physical Cures and Treatments

These are some examples of physical cures and treatments:

- ❖ Surgery
- ❖ Physical therapy
- ❖ Chiropractic care
- ❖ Exercise (rehab)
- ❖ Acupuncture

A doctor can treat you physically through surgery, in which organs or other body parts may be removed/

repaired. Alternatively, a patient may choose chiropractic care, physical therapy, rehabilitation, and acupuncture as other modes of physical care. All forms of care are directed at treating the physical side of health. Therefore, surgeons, chiropractic physicians, physical therapists, and acupuncturists treat the body physically. Although surgery at times may be necessary, it is not the way to improve your health. Removing organs, glands, joints, and nerves does not improve the function of the body; it weakens it. Through the other forms of care you can, in most instances, reduce the chances of surgery. Keeping your body parts is better than losing them, wouldn't you agree? So, although surgery may be necessary, it is a final line of defense. This is not the best time to deal with a problem, especially if you have ignored your condition for years. There's a well-known saying of Ben Franklin's: "An ounce of prevention is worth a pound of cure." Through chiropractic therapy, acupuncture, physical therapy, and exercise, you can reduce the risk of surgery and improve the health of the physical body. These therapies will be discussed at great length in the physical section of this book.

Mental/Emotional Cures and Treatment
Mental/Emotional Forms of Treatment Include:

❖ Psychiatry
❖ Psychology
❖ Medication
❖ Surgery
❖ Self-help books/tapes/seminars
❖ Religion

Although we need the branches of psychiatry and psychology, the majority of our society is made up of able people. I did not say we were perfect, but the majority of society can function in today's world. The majority of society would benefit from self-help books, DVDs, courses, or spiritual/religious self-education. These people could prosper on their own while enhancing their lives. By the way, this portion of society consists of the successful people you read, see, and hear about. They know how to apply life's principles, seizing and enjoying every moment on this earth. Now this skill would be of great benefit to the majority of society. This book will help guide and educate you in this endeavor. The secrets of successful people are all revealed in the mental/emotional section of achieving unlimited health. For what would life be without success?

So now, you understand that:

* The body has an inborn mechanism to survive and heal itself.
* The cause, cure, and treatment of all health problems are chemical, physical, and mental/emotional entities.
* Treating a chemical problem with anything other than the right chemical solution is suicide.
* Treating a physical problem with anything other than the right physical solution is suicide.
* Treating a mental/emotional problem with anything other than the right mental solution is suicide.
* Each side of your health has a dramatic influence on the other two sides of the triune. Therefore, a

12

You Are a Product of What You Eat

D id you know that your body is constantly repairing and rebuilding itself every six to twelve months? That's right! Every six to twelve months,

> *Let us prolong the regeneration of youth rather than perpetuate the degeneration of cancer and heart disease.*

you have a brand-new body. Every cell in the body is repaired or reproduced to maintain your survival. In fact, as Dr. Arthur C. Guyton states in his widely used *Textbook of Medical Physiology*, cells could live indefinitely, provided that "the surrounding fluids remain constant." Through nutrition, you can create the proper environment to keep the surrounding fluids constant. If this is done and you meet the nutritional demands of the body, then you should look and feel better six months to a year from now. If you do not give the body what it needs, you will age and feel worse than you do now. It is your choice. Do you want to grow old and rot on the vine or mature like a fine wine?

When I was young, in my twenties, people said that I was maturing. When I hit forty, people threw me an over-the-hill party. Do you see how that viewpoint can make you old before your time? Listen up. Your body hits its stride between the ages of forty and seventy. Your body should feel like the body of a fifteen- or sixteen-year-old, and you should have a healthy, matured look about you. People should compliment you on how great you look, regardless of your age. In fact, they should be amazed.

Our bodies are constantly repairing and making new cells at a rate of five million every five minutes. There are approximately one hundred trillion cells that make up the human body. The raw materials that your body requires to make these cells and the chemicals they produce come from the food you eat. If you eat junk food, your body feels and looks like junk. You are what you eat. Therefore, if the raw materials that you need to build a new cell are present when the cell is being created, you are creating the best possible environment to build a cell that is healthier than the one it is replacing. If you don't give your body the proper nourishment, you cause continued cell damage, leading to malfunction, disease, and finally symptoms. When you build a house, do you go to a building-supply company, or do you go to a junkyard? If you take pride in the building of your home, then why not take pride in the building of your body? If you do not take care of your body, where else are you going to live? Therefore, we can chemically enhance our health through nutrition. The foods we eat today become part of us tomorrow—that is a scary thought for some.

Most everyone agrees on the importance of nutrition, but beyond that, there is much disagreement about what

> *Let the body mature like a fine wine rather than rot on the vine.*

constitutes healthy food. Taking nutrition seriously will alter the destiny of your life. This book will guide you systematically in creating your own signature nutritional program. Nutrition is a very serious and confusing topic for most people. In fact, the more you know, the more confused you become, due to the immensity of the subject matter. I will give you the 20 percent of what you are required to know about nutrition, which will give you 80 percent of your results. In this book, I have taken the confusion out of nutrition so that you can apply these principles to your daily regimen. In fact, the less you know, the easier it will be to follow these principles:

{ If you do not take care of your body, where else are you going to live? }

- ❖ Step 1. Determine what types of food you should eat. Should you eat meat, dairy, and fish, or are beans a better source of protein? Is wine OK? How about ice cream? Is pasta better than rice, etc.?
- ❖ Step 2. Clean up your diet to reduce chemical oxidants and chemically damaged (processed) foods.
- ❖ Step 3. Determine your optimum caloric, protein, fat, and carbohydrate intakes.
- ❖ Step 4. Determine what supplements you need to take, understanding why they are necessary in today's society.

Once you complete these steps, you will have come a long way. In six months to a year, you will notice a new you—younger, more vibrant, healthier, and happier. If that prospect doesn't excite you, nothing will.

Let's get started on our journey. The information in this book explains why, how, and what you need to succeed. I will keep my explanations brief and simple. Let's start with the composition of food, which will help us with the first step.

All foods contain a combination of proteins, fats, and carbohydrates. Most foods contain high amounts of either proteins or fats or carbohydrates. For example, pasta is loaded with carbohydrates, whereas lean meat is loaded with protein. The yolk of an egg is cholesterol (fat), and the egg white is all protein.

Why should we know this? Proteins, carbohydrates, and fats serve a purpose to the health of the body. This is what we will explore next. In the meanwhile, look at the chart on the next page to find out which foods are considered carbohydrates, proteins, or fats. Please note that most, if not all, food is a combination of all three.

The Composition of Food

All Foods Fall under These Three Headings

Carbohydrates
Grains
Wheat, rice, oats, barley,
Rye bread, pasta, and cereals

Vegetables
High-fiber, low-starch
Leafy greens: lettuce, cabbage, spinach
Seeded: tomatoes and cucumbers
Stalks/shoots: celery, sprouts, mushrooms

Low-fiber, high-starch (sugar)
Potatoes, corn, carrots, beets
Legumes (high protein)
Beans, peas, lentils
Beans, Peas and Lentils

Fruits
High-sugar
Fruit juices: apple and orange
Dried fruits: raisins and figs

Low/medium-sugar
Melons: watermelons and cantelopes
Citrus: oranges and lemons
Cherries and berries: black, blue, red
Processed carbohydrates
Cakes, candy, soda, alcohol

Proteins
Red meat
Flank, sirloin, brisket, veal

Fowl
Chicken and turkey

Fish/shell
Tuna, lobster, flounder

Dairy
Milk, eggs, cheese

Nuts/seeds
Almonds and cashews

Legumes
Beans, peas, lentils

Processed
Salami, bologna, frankfurters

Fats
Red meat

Fowl

Fish/shell

Dairy

Nuts/seeds

Oils
Olive and sesame

Processed

13

The Purpose of Carbohydrates, Fats, and Proteins

N ow that you know the composition of food, let's look at why each one is important to health. The purpose of food in general is to give your body the raw materials it needs to:

❖ Repair and rebuild your cells. Proteins and fats are used to rebuild your cells.
❖ Produce all the chemicals (blood, antibodies, hormones, and enzymes) necessary for survival. Again, proteins and fats are used to produce the majority of these chemicals produced by the body.
❖ Produce energy to run all bodily processes, such as digestion, thought, muscular contraction, breathing, etc. In this case, carbohydrates, fats, and proteins are used for energy.

Now that we know the purpose of food, let's touch on each of the three above. As far as importance goes, protein is ranked number one, fat number two, and carbohydrate number three. In other words, when determining your nutritional regimen, your protein source quality and quantity will be the most important followed by fat and carbohydrates. Unfortunately, most people do the opposite.

Hierarchy of Food, with the Most Important First

1. Protein
2. Fat
3. Carbohydrate

Protein

After water, which makes up 50–70 percent of the human body, protein is the next most abundant substance. At 30–40 percent, it makes up your muscles, bones, nerves, organs/glands, and skin. The name was coined by the Dutch chemist, Gerard Johann Mulder (1838), meaning "of the first importance." People make me laugh when they concern themselves with the right type of vitamin or mineral and never stop to think about protein intake. The amount of protein is important, but the type and quality of the protein you eat is equally important. Protein is necessary in the repair and rebuilding of your body. Protein makes up all chemical production mentioned above and can be converted into carbohydrates and fat by the body to use as energy. Please note that fat and carbohydrate cannot be converted into protein by the body. Protein is used to literally regenerate the body. Without a sufficient amount of daily protein, your body cannot regenerate itself. Lacking protein, your body enters a degenerative phase. If the body does not receive its daily protein requirement, it robs Peter to pay Paul. In other words, it pulls protein from another part of your body that needs it less than the area that needs it now. This will cause chemical and cellular damage, leading to diseases, such as cancer and heart disease. I always like to say protein is the backbone of your embodiment.

Determining your protein requirement is an absolute must, since your nutritional program will evolve around it. (This will be discussed in detail later in this section.) Again, if I had to choose the most important of the three (carbohydrate, fat, protein), it would have to be protein. Protein, in almost all cases, are found in the same foods as fat. So, by eating a proper amount of protein, you will get your fat requirement.

Fat

If protein serves as your body's bricks, fat is its cement. When building a brick building, you need mortar (cement) so that the bricks adhere to each other. Most people do not realize the importance of fat and look at its downside. Here are the reasons why fat is important in our diets:

1. Fat, in conjunction with protein, produces cells and body chemicals. In nature, fat and protein are always found together, so it stands to reason that your body requires both together. I think God intended it to be that way since she/he created the food in the first place.
2. Fat is also responsible for the production of cell membranes, hormones, enzymes, and antibodies.
3. Fat protects and cushions your organs.

4. Fat acts as an insulator for your nervous system and skin, preventing nerves from short circuiting and regulating heat and water loss through the skin.
5. Fat is a primary component in the production of lymph. Lymph, as you may know, acts as the body's sanitation system, carrying away cellular debris, metabolic wastes, etc.
6. Fat is used for energy and heat production (metabolic stimulation).

This is why we crave fat: it is precious. We need fat. I repeat: We need fat. Stop this low-fat/no-fat trash. It is not healthy!

Carbohydrate

Carbohydrates are used for energy, which can be instant or stored. This energy is necessary to run all bodily processes. Please note that carbohydrates are not the raw materials that produce cells but only the energy necessary to make and fuel them. There are very few cellular structures made with carbohydrates, but importantly the DNA molecule is one of them. Carbohydrates are also converted and stored as fat. So taking in too many carbohydrates can lead to obesity, just as eating too much fat can.

Water

Your body is 50–75 percent water. Water is a universal solvent, which means all body chemicals have to be able to react with one another in a water solution. Water also acts as a transport system, and is the medium used for all chemical reactions and metabolic processes. The term "wet fire" is appropriate when discussing the role of water in metabolism for the above reasons. So, my first priority is water intake.

Before figuring out your foods (proteins, fats, and carbohydrates), focus on water, especially between meals since it curbs appetite and is the greatest appetite suppressant I know. Please note, I did not say juice, coffee, wine, beer, soda—I said water. Water is also necessary to take fat out of storage. When fat is stored in the body, a molecule of water is cleaved (separated) from the fat to reduce storage space. When the fat is ready to be used again by the body, the water molecule has to be added back to the fat. So by drinking more water you will lose more fat. Water helps cleanse and detoxify the body of metabolic wastes and excessive minerals and salts. If I had to choose the type of water (tap, bottled, distilled etc.) I would choose reverse osmosis, and this is why:

1. Removes all impurities, odors, and contaminants.
2. Tastes great and makes coffee or tea or whatever you cook taste better (soups/pasta/oatmeal).
3. Can use with pets, plants, and aquariums.
4. Much less expensive than bottled water.

The amount of water that you should take in varies based on many factors, such as water loss from exercise or work, but as a general rule of thumb, it should be about one-fourth to one-half ounce of water per pound of lean body weight. So, if your lean body weight is 150 pounds, you should be taking in between one and two quarts per day between meals, as a minimum. Drink more if you are physically active or sweat a lot due to climate. Another good rule of thumb is to look at the color of your urine, which should be a pale yellow color from a pigment called urochrome. That color normally varies from pale yellow to deep amber, depending on the concentration of the urine. Darker urine is usually a sign that you're not drinking enough fluid. So if you notice the color of your urine growing darker and you are urinating less, it would be a fair assumption that you are dehydrating or, worse yet, dehydrated.

The Effects of Dehydration

We rarely pay attention to how a decrease in water intake can damage our body. It is estimated that 75 percent of Americans are chronically dehydrated. The brain is composed of between 85–92 percent water, and a loss of even 1 percent leads to irreversible damage. As you can see, keeping the brain well hydrated is very important.

A study done titled "The effects of dehydration on brain volume" by Dickson JM et al. in the department of biomedical science at the University of Sheffield noted the following:

1. Mild dehydration leads to an increase in your appetite, and you confuse thirst with hunger.
2. Mild dehydration can slow down your metabolism by 3 percent.
3. 1 percent dehydration leads to thirst.

4. 2 percent dehydration causes feelings of anxiety, reduced appetite, and a decrease in strength and capacity for work by 20 percent.
5. 4 percent dehydration brings feelings of nausea, dizziness, emotional instability, and fatigue.
6. 6 percent dehydration leads to loss of coordination and coherence of speech.
7. 10 percent dehydration causes thermoregulation (cannot maintain body temperature) failure in addition to all above mentioned symptoms. Cells begin to die.
8. At 11 percent dehydration, it's not enough just to drink water. The chemical balance of the organism has undergone serious changes. In order to restore it, you need professional medical care.
9. 20 percent dehydration may lead to death.

Major Symptoms of Dehydration

❖ Exhaustion, lack of energy
❖ Constipation
❖ Eating disorders
❖ Low or high blood pressure
❖ Gastritis, gastric ulcer
❖ Problems with the respiratory system
❖ Improper acid-alkaline balance
❖ Extra weight and obesity
❖ Eczema
❖ High cholesterol
❖ Cystitis, infections of the urinary canal
❖ Joint, muscle ache and pain, as well as rheumatism

Signs of Dehydration in Children

- ❖ Sunken eyes
- ❖ Decreased frequency of urination or dry diapers
- ❖ Sunken soft spot on the front of the head in babies (called the fontanel)
- ❖ No tears when the child cries
- ❖ Dry or sticky mucous membranes (the lining of the mouth or tongue)
- ❖ Lethargy (less than normal activity)
- ❖ Irritability

Now that you know the three food groups and the importance of water, let's discuss the importance of quality. You want to make sure that the quality of your protein, fat, and carbohydrates are USDA Grade A. When you put fuel into your high-performance car, you don't use el cheapo gas, do you? You should not treat your body any differently.

14

Quality Food Groups

Before you figure out what types of food are good for you, I would like to jump ahead and first explain how we damage our foods. Let's take each food group and explain how processing can damage the quality of that particular food. Then we will discuss ways to help clean up this portion of your diet.

Carbohydrates

Carbohydrates are damaged in many ways. When you grow carbohydrates (fruits, vegetables, and grains), damage can occur from pesticides and other poisonous substances used to deter insects, birds, and rodents from eating the food. Although pesticides protect the food from insects, they act as a poison to us and can cause chemical damage, especially to our nervous systems.

Using synthetic fertilizers and not giving soil back the nutrients that previously grown crops have depleted reduces the vitamin and mineral content in the foods grown. In fact, there are studies that emphasize this very point. They estimate that mineral and vitamin content in foods grown today are only 40 to 60 percent of what they were forty to fifty years ago. Therefore, we have to take in twice the amount of food to get the same amount of vitamins and minerals. However, taking in twice the amount of food doubles our caloric intake, which leads to obesity.

The processing of natural sugars through pasteurization, such as with milk sugar (lactose), can damage the molecular structure of the sugar, leading to lactose intolerance. The processing of converting cane (brown sugar) into white sugar removes what is left of the natural vitamins and minerals found in cane sugar, giving you an empty-calorie food. The only thing left in these foods after processing is calories—with no or low vitamin and mineral content. This leads to rapid increases in blood sugar, because the sugar enters your bloodstream immediately, creating mood swings that can lead to hyperactivity, anxiety, and depression. Often this is accompanied by rapid weight gain due to the storage of this excess sugar as fat.

The processing of grains (starches), such as those found in breads, pasta, rice, and cereals, also depletes the vitamin and mineral content. Again, the calories remain, which lead to obesity. These refined starches also act as allergens, creating the so-called "gluten reactions," which cause immediate, excessive mucous production in the digestive tract and sinuses. Genetically engineered grains are gaining popularity with the big food companies but will cause many problems when our body is faced with the utilization of these genetically mutated foods.

The process of distillation (concentrates) has a similar reaction on the chemical structure of fruit and can turn fruit, potatoes or grain into alcohol, which in excessive/concentrated amounts can be highly toxic to the liver.

The process of preserving food with chemicals to prevent spoilage also depletes nutrients. Oxidation is a fancy term for food spoilage. For example, if you leave food out on the table uncovered, it spoils faster than if it were in the freezer. This is due to the outside air (oxidation, meaning "with oxygen") and warm temperature, which together accelerate microbial action. The oxygen in the air causes evaporation, burning off the vitamins and minerals in the food in the process. Therefore, to retard oxidation, manufacturers use chemicals known as preservatives that attach themselves to the vitamin/mineral portion of the food, preventing their release when food is exposed to oxygen. The only problem is that these bound-up vitamins and minerals are not released when the food is eaten, rendering them useless to us while causing a toxic reaction to the body due to the preservative.

Food dyes and additives designed to enhance taste/color only heighten this craziness by increasing your appetite. By consuming moderate to excessive amounts of additives, which are highly addictive, we further deplete the vitamin and mineral content in the food as we become addicted to these foods. What makes matters worse is that now, when these preservatives enter your body, your body must neutralize, destroy, or rid itself of these harmful substances. To do this, the body requires enzymes, antibodies, and hormones, which contain the precious vitamins and minerals in reserve that we must now use to counter the effects of all these toxic chemicals. Therefore, we put little in and take a lot out. So then, how do we improve the quality of our carbohydrates? Below is a list of things that you can do immediately:

1. Use fresh or frozen fruits and vegetables (make sure you clean and wash all). These have no chemical preservatives, additives, salts, and colorings. Canned goods and processed dinners contain higher levels of these chemical ingredients. These chemicals increase food toxicity and decrease vitamin and mineral content.
2. Use whole grains instead of white flour. This increases the vitamin and mineral content. The white flour also creates a heightened gluten reaction, which I already mentioned. This leads to food allergies as well as other sinus conditions.
3. Use natural sweeteners: cane (brown), fruit, milk, and honey instead of white sugar products. These foods have higher vitamin and mineral levels.
4. Do not use artificial sweeteners that only heighten your taste for sweetness. Eventually even sugar does not taste sweet, making you add more sugar to your coffee, leading to obesity.
5. Buy organically grown foods when you can. These vegetables and fruits have higher vitamin and mineral content, and you will avoid pesticides and chemical fertilizers, thereby reducing the toxic effects on your body.

Protein

Protein is damaged by the contamination of our streams and rivers, which affect our fish. They are also damaged through the hormones given to our chickens and cows. Additives, preservatives, coloring, flavoring, as well as increased fat concentration in the meat is why people frown upon meat. So follow the rules below to improve the quality of your protein intake.

1. Stay away from luncheon meats (bologna, salami, sausage, liverwurst, franks, and beef jerky). This will dramatically reduce your fat content as well as your salts, nitrates, and nitrites leading to water retention.
2. If you are concerned about hormones, do not eat the skin or visible fat on meat or fowl, since the hormonal residue is stored mostly in the fat. If you want to further avoid hormones, you could purchase range-fed beef, which is free of hormones.
3. Sources of protein: below are what I consider the more important sources of protein, due to the higher percentage of protein in the food. This is followed by secondary sources that supplement the meal, completing the balance.

Primary sources of protein:

❖ Lean cuts of meat (beef, veal, lamb, pork, and wild game)
❖ Fowl (chicken, turkey, duck, and wild game)
❖ Fish and egg whites

Secondary sources of protein:

❖ Dairy (cheese, milk)
❖ Beans (soy, black, lima, etc.)
❖ Grains (wheat, rye, rice)

4. If you use packaged, mixed, or canned protein drinks, keep them to a minimum.

Nothing works like Mother Nature. Remember, you must first balance your protein intake. This will give you the fat intake, which will determine your carbohydrates. This will be discussed under the quantity section. Choose any of the protein listed on the table of foods, choosing the primary proteins in your diet first. Then choose your secondary proteins to help fill in the gaps. This is the new paradigm shift: focus on protein first, then fat, and then carbohydrates. How to assess which types of protein to eat and how much will be discussed later.

Fat

Avoid fat that is hydrogenated (fat that is bombarded with hydrogen); they are almost impossible for the body to utilize correctly and only clog up body chemistry. Most hydrogenated fats (trans fats) are found in most of your processed foods and make the food taste better, making you eat more.

Follow the principles below to improve the quality of your fat intake.

1. Stay away from (or reduce to a minimum of one or two days a week) all luncheon meats, as mentioned in the protein section.
2. Care must be given when buying store/restaurant cakes, pies, chips, hamburgers, or anything cooked in fat or with fat added. These foods usually contain a lot of hydrogenated oils and fat.

3. Avoid processed, low-fat foods. Although they are low in fat, they contain a lot of chemical alteration and high carbohydrate levels.
4. If you eat the proper amount and type of protein, you will get the proper amount of fat.

This is a basic overview of how you can immediately clean up your diet. Following these steps will give your body the necessary raw materials to repair and rebuild itself properly. At this point, we have a good sense about what we want to do. To make the next step simple, I have a list of what I consider healthy foods. All you have to do is get a pen/yellow marker and check all the things you want to eat or enjoy eating.

Pretend you are in your favorite restaurant and you are picking out your favorite dishes. What would they be? This is fun. Do not laugh, because you are about to design your own nutritional profile program. Once you pick these foods, I will show you how to combine them to create mouth-watering, healthy meals.

Before you start to pick your foods, please follow the principles below:

❖ When picking your food, pick foods that you really enjoy, regardless of what you think. What is your favorite breakfast, lunch, and dinner? Let your decision come from your intuition.

❖ Look at your heritage. Speak to your parents and grandparents about what was eaten in the old country. For generations, over thousands of years, diets and heritage changed little in most cultures around the world. They ate what was grown, gathered, or hunted; therefore, from a genetic point of view, your ancestors had many generations to adapt to those foods. During the last three or four generations, we experienced a dramatic culture shock as far as nutrition is concerned. You can be whisked around the globe in hours. Thanks to refrigeration, transportation, and processed food, you can eat American in the morning, Chinese at lunch, and Italian for dinner. We also have more chemicals in our food than we have in the chemical makeup of that food. Our bodies have not had time to adapt genetically or biochemically to this rapid chemical change. Genetically, our bodies have undergone chemical genetic damage, due to these rapid dietary changes. So, if at all possible, please determine your heritage, because the foods eaten in your culture are best suited for you from a genetic, biochemical point of view.

If you are still not sure, a fasting blood chemistry (SMAC/25, CBC/DIFF, and urinalysis) can be used with the above criteria to accurately assess your nutritional needs. For more information about this test and how you can have it performed, please contact my office at 561-627-3810, or you can e-mail me at drcima@cimahealth.com
What are you waiting for? Pick your foods,
and have fun!

15

Food Calorie/Percentage Charts

Meat/Fowl

2 oz. Serving	Total Calories	Fat Calories	% of Fat	Protein Calories	% of Protein
Tenderloin	190	135	70	55	30
Rib eye	170	110	65	60	35
T-bone	170	110	65	60	35
Porterhouse	170	110	65	60	35
Brisket	170	65	35	105	65
Ground	160	80	50	80	50
Flank	140	70	50	70	50
Sirloin	115	40	35	75	65
Bacon	75	25	30	50	70
Lamb	150	90	60	60	70
Kabob	80	32	40	48	60
Veal	70	15	30	55	80
Venison	70	15	20	55	80
Duck w/skin	230	207	90	23	10
Duck w/o skin	70	31	45	39	55
Chicken w/skin	120	72	60	48	40

2 oz. Serving	Total Calories	Fat Calories	% of Fat	Protein Calories	% of Protein
Chicken w/o skin	70	21	30	49	70
Turkey w/skin	90	45	50	45	50
Turkey w/o skin	65	20	30	45	70

Nuts and Oils

2 oz. Serving	Total Calories	Fat Calories	% of Fat
Nuts			
Almonds	360	270	75
Cashews	300	240	80
Peanuts	320	270	80
Brazil nuts	370	320	85
Pecans	360	325	90
Walnuts	350	315	90
Oils			
Canola, sesame	500	500	100
Vegetable	500	500	100
Corn, olive	500	500	100
Soybean, sunflower	500	500	100

Fish

2 oz. Serving	Total Calories	Fat Calories	% of Fat	Protein Calories	% of Protein
Pompano	100	50	50	50	50
Salmon	80	40	50	40	50
Sardines	120	60	50	60	50
Trout	85	42	50	43	50

2 oz. Serving	Total Calories	Fat Calories	% of Fat	Protein Calories	% of Protein
Tuna (oil)	110	55	50	55	50
Whitefish	75	33	50	37	50
Mackerel	120	60	50	60	50
Sea trout	60	18	30	42	70
Tuna (blue fin)	80	25	30	55	70
Bluefish	70	20	30	50	70
Catfish	70	20	30	50	70
Tilefish	50	10	20	40	80

2 oz. Serving	Total Calories	Fat Calories to Protein Calories
Clams	40	<10% of calories >90% of calories
Cod	45	<10% of calories >90% of calories
Crab, Alaskan	50	<10% of calories >90% of calories
Dolphin	50	<10% of calories >90% of calories
Flounder	50	<10% of calories >90% of calories
Grouper	50	<10% of calories >90% of calories
Haddock	50	<10% of calories >90% of calories
Halibut	60	<10% of calories >90% of calories
Perch	50	<10% of calories >90% of calories
Pike—Northern	50	<10% of calories >90% of calories
Scallops	50	<10% of calories >90% of calories
Sea bass	50	<10% of calories >90% of calories
Shrimp	60	<10% of calories >90% of calories
Tarpon	50	<10% of calories >90% of calories
Tuna (water)	80	<10% of calories >90% of calories

Legumes, Beans, and Peas

2 oz. Serving	Total Calories	Grams Protein/ Grams Carbs	Grams Protein/ Calories
Mung	190	14/56	36/145
Lima	190	12/48	36/145
Pinto	190	12/48	36/145
Soybean	90	8/32	7/280
Black bean	180	12/48	36/145
Black-eye	80	10/24	16/64
Adzuki	190	11/45	36/145
Navy	190	13/52	35/140
Lentil	70	5/20	13/52
Split pea	200	14/56	34/136

Dairy

Dairy Product	Total Calories	Fat Calories	% of Fat	Protein Calories	% of Protein
Eggs					
Large egg	75	60 (yolk)	80	15	20
Lg. egg white	15	0	0	15	100
Milk (2 fl. oz.)					
Skim	24	2	<10	22	0
Low-fat 1%	24	6	2	18	75
Low-fat 2%	30	9	30	21	70
Whole milk	36	18	50	18	50
Cheese (2 oz.)					
Cottage, low-fat	50	10	20	40	80

Dairy Product	Total Calories	Fat Calories	% of Fat	Protein Calories	% of Protein
Cottage, regular	60	36	60	24	30
Feta	150	90	60	60	40
Mozzarella	180	100	60	80	40
Ricotta	100	60	60	40	40
Romano	200	120	60	80	40
Provolone	200	120	60	80	40
Parmesan	200	120	60	80	40
Swiss	200	120	60	80	40
American	200	160	80	40	20
Blue	200	160	80	40	20
Brick	200	160	80	40	20
Brie	200	160	80	40	20
Camembert	170	130	80	40	20
Cheddar	228	180	80	48	20
Limburger	200	160	80	40	20
Monterey Jack	200	160	80	40	20
Butter (2 oz.)					
½ stick	400	400	100	0	0
Whipped	270	270	100	0	0

Grains

2 oz. Serving	Total Calories	Fat Calories	% of Fat
Barley	200	<10% fat	
Buckwheat	200		<10
Wheat	200		<10
Wheat bran	120	24	20
Wheat flour	200		<10
Wheat germ	200	60	30
Cornmeal	200		
Corn starch	200		
Corn gain	200		
Corn grits	200		
Millet	200		<10
Oats	220	35	15
Oat bran	140	35	25
Bran	200	40	20
Rice			
2 oz. uncooked	200		
Rice cake	60		
2 oz. rye	190		

Vegetables

2 oz. Serving	Total Calories
Celery	10
Cucumber	10
Endive	10
Lemon	10
Lettuce	10
Radish	10
Sauerkraut	10
Swiss chard	10
Tomatoes, green or red	10
Zucchini	10
Asparagus	15
Broccoli	15
Cabbage	15
Cauliflower	15
Eggplant	15
Mushroom	15
Pepper, green or red	15
Spinach	15
Turnips	15
Beets	20
Green beans	20
Lime	20
Onion	20
Rutabaga	20

2 oz. Serving	Total Calories
Squash	20
Vegetable juice	30
Brussels sprouts	30
Butternut squash	30
Carrot	30
Carrot juice	30
Kale	30
Corn	35
Fig	40
Green peas	40

2 oz. Serving	Total Calories	Total Fat
Tofu	45	50
Tomato paste/potato	50	
Sweet potato/water chestnut	60	
Avocado (Florida)	60	66
Yams	66	
Avocado (California)	90	80
Olive	100	90

Fruit

2 oz. Serving	Total Calories
Cantaloupe	20
Grapefruit	20
Honeydew	20
Strawberry	20

2 oz. Serving	Total Calories
Watermelon	20
Banana, peeled	25
Orange, peeled	25
Peach, pitted	25
Tangerine	25
Apple juice	30
Blackberry	30
Blueberry	30
Cherry	30
Cranberry	30
Orange	30
Raspberry	30
Plum	30
Nectarine	30
Pineapple	30
Apple	35
Cherry juice	35
Pear	35
Grapes	35
Pineapple juice	35
Grape juice	40
Apple cider	45

16

Quantity of Food

Now that you have a quality diet, quantity becomes our major focus. How do you combine your food at meal times and know approximately how much to eat? Simply following the points outlined below. When you design any meal, first ask yourself what your protein is going to be. The reason for this was addressed earlier, but I will review it again. In addition to water, the body is mostly made up of protein and fat. Proteins can be converted into fats as well as sugars (carbs). In reality, protein can make fat and sugar. The same cannot be said for fat and sugar, since each cannot manufacture protein. The main reason you crave food is due to this protein deficiency in your nutritional profile. Therefore, you know that you need protein.

Below are things you must know, understand, and use in your nutritional profile.

❖ 1 gram of protein = 4 calories.
❖ 1 gram of carbohydrate = 4 calories.
❖ 1 gram of fat = 9 calories.
❖ 28 grams of protein, carbohydrates, or fat = 1 ounce.

❖ 1 ounce of protein or carbohydrate =112 (28x4) calories.
❖ 1 ounce of fat = 252 (28x9) calories.

Please take your time reading this section, and read it many times if need be.
This is a one-time process, and once you complete the calculations you are golden.

Rule 1

Your protein intake should be a minimum of one gram per pound of lean body weight. If your lean weight is 150 pounds, you would need to take in a minimum of 150 grams of protein daily, or about five ounces (150/28 (grams in one ounce) = 5.3). If you are not sure what your lean weight is, just look at what you weigh now and what you think you should weigh. Let's be realistic and not go back to when you were in high school and weighed a hundred pounds if you now weigh two hundred pounds. In this case, I would use 150 pounds of lean weight for now. Please note that when I say five ounces of protein, I do not mean portion size. I mean pure protein. Most people think that when they eat five ounces of fish, they are getting five ounces of protein. When you eat five ounces of fish, you are getting about one ounce of protein. The list below explains why:

❖ 6 ounces of red meat gives you 2–3.5 ounces of protein (10–70 percent fat).
❖ 6 ounces of fowl gives you 1–2.5 ounces of protein (30 percent fat without skin, 60 percent with skin).

❖ 6 ounces of cheese gives you 1.5–2 ounces of protein (60–80 percent fat).

❖ 6 ounces of fish gives you 1–1.5 ounces of protein (10–50 percent fat).

❖ 6 ounces of egg whites gives you 1 ounce of protein (0 percent fat).

❖ 6 ounces of cooked beans gives you one-fourth to one-half ounce of protein (50–75 percent carbohydrates).

A specific breakdown of each protein for fat content is listed in the table of food, and can be found on the internet as well.

Now you can better see why I choose meats, fowl, fish, and egg whites as primary proteins, since they have the highest protein-to-fat ratio. They are either rich sources of protein or have a high protein-efficiency ratio (proteins that are easily digested by the body), as in the case of egg whites, or have moderate to low amounts of fat. Therefore, by using the formula above, you can now calculate your body's protein needs and eat what you want from the list above to fulfill your requirements.

Rule 2

Follow the next two steps to find the number of calories you should be taking in. Most people starve themselves by not eating enough calories. By the way, the fastest way to become obese is to starve yourself. Remember this statement:

{ *Just like your car, if you want to speed up your metabolism, you give your body more of the right fuel and not less of the wrong fuel. Now that's powerful* }

1. You must estimate your daily caloric intake. To estimate your total caloric intake, follow this formula:

   ❖ Take your lean weight or the weight you want to be, and be realistic. Now multiply that number by 10.
   ❖ If your lean weight or desired weight was 150, then your caloric intake is 150 x 10 = 1,500 calories.
      ❖ This represents (approximately), the *minimal daily caloric intake* that your body needs to function or what we call your *basal metabolic rate*.

2. Determine your *metabolic accelerator rate*. There are three activity levels that you can put yourself in: sedentary, moderate, or active.

   ❖ <u>Sedentary</u>: A person who does not exercise and does little, if any, physical work or activity. Multiply your caloric intake by 25 percent.
   ❖ <u>Moderate</u>: A person who exercises three to four hours (moderate intensity) per week or has a moderately physically demanding job (housewife/mother). Multiply your caloric intake by 50 percent.
   ❖ <u>Active</u>: A person who exercises six or more hours (intensely) per week or has a physically demanding job, such as construction/labor. Multiply your caloric intake by 75–100 percent. Please note athletes may require much more protein.

So, if you weigh 150 pounds and lead a moderately active lifestyle, your caloric intake should range from 1,500 to 2,250:
- ❖ *150 x 10 = 1,500*
- ❖ *1,500 x 50 percent (moderate lifestyle) = 750*
- ❖ *1,500 + 750 = 2,250*

Rule 3

Follow the next steps to determine your protein requirements.

1. To calculate your protein requirements:

    - ❖ Take your weight or desired weight and divide that number by 28 (there are 28 grams in one ounce of protein).
    - ❖ This gives you your *minimum ounces of protein.*

For example, if you weigh 150 pounds, you would divide 150 by 28, which would give you the number of ounces of protein (minimum) that you will need. In this case, it is approximately 5.3 or (rounded off to the nearest ounce) 5 ounces of protein.

2. Now add your activity level to the figure above, which gives you your maximum protein requirement.

    - ❖ Sedentary: no extra protein
    - ❖ Moderate: two ounces of extra protein
    - ❖ Active: three to four ounces of extra protein

Using the above example of 150 pounds having a moderate activity level would require seven ounces of protein each day (5+2 for moderate activity).

3. Multiply the above two numbers by 28 (this gives you the total number of grams of protein).

   ❖ *Five ounces gives you 5x28=140 grams of protein*
   ❖ *Seven ounces gives you 7 x28=196 grams of protein*

4. Then multiply each number by four (four calories per gram). This gives you your minimum/maximum protein caloric intake.

   ❖ *Five ounces=140 grams x 4 calories =560 calories to*
   ❖ *Seven ounces=196 grams x 4 calories= 784 calories*

Please note: Once these numbers are calculated, you have the basics done. Please take the time to do the math now. It will be well worth your while, believe me! If you do not do this, you will either starve yourself or eat yourself to death with the wrong foods. Now, on a daily basis, you will use these numbers to determine how well you are eating on any given day. The steps below are to be performed on a daily basis. I know this is tough, but your health depends on it. Therefore, it's worth three minutes of your time.

Rule 4

You must estimate your fat intake. Your protein caloric intake = your fat caloric intake. *For example, suppose you took in five hundred calories of protein. Your fat calories would also be five hundred calories.* Please note that this is an estimate, based on what I believe is a balanced protein-to-fat ratio from primary and secondary sources of protein that I mentioned earlier (see below). If you eat the various primary and secondary sources of protein, you will average a fat intake of 25–35 percent. Remember each gram of fat equals nine calories. If you want to be as accurate as possible, you can use the table of foods I have included to get accurate percentages of fat levels, but this is not necessary.

Primary sources of protein:
Lean cuts of meat (beef, veal, lamb, and wild game)
Fowl (chicken, turkey, duck, and wild game)
Fish and egg whites

Secondary sources of protein:
Dairy (cheese, milk)

Beans (soy, black, lima, etc.)

Rule 5

You must estimate your carbohydrate intake. To determine the amount of carbohydrates you can eat each day, subtract your total protein and fat caloric intake from your total calories.

For example, a 150-pound person with a moderate lifestyle would need between 1500-2,250 calories per day.

- *The protein intake for this person would be about seven ounces of protein*
- *Each ounce of protein =112 calories x seven ounces of protein = 784 calories or let's say 800 calories.*
- *This is also your caloric intake of fat. Therefore, the total caloric intake is 800 calories from protein and 800 calories from fat totaling 1,600 calories.*
- *Now subtract 1,600 calories from the maximum calorie intake of 2,250 calories, gives you your carbohydrate intake, which is 650 calories. That 650 calories in carbohydrates is equivalent to three to four ounces of pasta, plus one to two slices of bread, a four-ounce serving of veggies, and two ounces of fruit. Or if you want to have more fruit and veggies decrease the pasta or bread slightly. Now that's what I call a nutritional program!*

Therefore, you start your meal with a fatty protein and then combine the right amount of carbohydrate calories to round out the meal. Remember, the leaner the protein, the more carbohydrates you can have. You must also know which carbohydrates to combine with which proteins. The wrong combinations can be deadly. This process is known as food combining, which I will discuss next. This is very important, since food combining impacts digestive success.

Before I address food combining, there is a worksheet on the next page. Please take the time to fill it out. This will give you a good idea of portion control and how many calories, how much protein, fat, and carbohydrate you really require. This will be the beginning of your journey, and if you plot it correctly, you will be reimbursed handsomely with an aesthetic, functional body that will defy the aging process as you mature gracefully. Never again will you feel guilty or deprive your body of what it truly requires. If you are truly looking for success, please take the time to fill this out.

Calorie Worksheet

1. Take your weight (or the weight you want to be) and multiply it by 10:

    _____ x 10 =_____
    Weight   Minimum daily caloric intake (Min.DCI)

2. Now take your activity level (sedentary: 25percent; moderate; 50 percent; or active: 75–100 percent). Multiply your minimum caloric intake by the right activity level.

    _____ x _____ % = _____
    Min. DCI   Activity

3. Add this number to your minimum daily caloric intake, which gives you your maximum daily intake.

    _____ + _____ = _____
    Min. DCI   Number2   Maximum daily caloric intake (MAX.DCI)

4. You now know your *caloric intake range*.
    Please write it down: _____-_____.
                         Min. DCI   Max. DCI

5. Divide your weight in pounds by 28.

    _____lbs./28 = _____oz.
    Weight   Minimum oz. of protein

6. Add your activity level to your minimum ounces of protein (sedentary: zero; moderate: two; active: two to four).

_____oz. + _____ = _____oz.

Min. protein   Activity   Maximum protein

7. Multiply the minimum and maximum ounces of protein by 28; this will give you the minimum and maximum grams of protein.

_____oz. x 28 =_____ grams   _____oz. x 28= _____ grams

Min. protein   Min. protein grams   Max. protein   Max. protein grams

8. Multiply the minimum and maximum grams of protein by four; this will give you the minimum and maximum caloric intake of protein.

_____ grams x 4 = _____ cal.   _____ grams x 4 = _____ cal.

Min. protein   Minimum caloric   Max. protein   Max. caloric

           intake of protein   intake of protein

9. Your protein caloric intake = your fat caloric intake:

_____ cal.   _____ cal.

Minimum fat caloric intake   Maximum fat caloric intake

10. Add your minimum fat caloric intake to your minimum protein caloric intake, and subtract from your minimum caloric intake:

11. _____ + _____ = _____
     Min. fat   Min. protein   Min. fat/protein calories
     caloric   caloric

12. _____ - _____ = _____
     Min. daily   Min. fat/protein Min. carbohydrate caloric intake
     caloric   caloric

13. Add your maximum fat caloric intake to your maximum protein caloric intake, and subtract from your maximum caloric intake:

14. _____ + _____ = _____
     Max. fat   Max. protein   Max. fat/protein calories
     caloric   caloric

15. _____ - _____ = _____
     Max. daily   Max. fat/   Max. carbohydrate caloric intake
     caloric   protein

16. Now you can fill in the chart below to help you decide how much to eat each day:

_____/_____Minimum/maximum daily caloric
                          intake

_____/_____Minimum/maximum oz. of protein (fat)

_____/_____Minimum/maximum grams of protein
                          (fat)

_____/_____Minimum/maximum calories of
protein

_____/_____Minimum/maximum calories of fat

_____/_____Minimum/maximum calories of
carbohydates

17

Food Combining

A major problem that I find with most people is that they do not combine food properly, which leads to digestive problems. Without going into too much detail, your stomach and digestive organs secrete enzymes to digest your food. Each type of food requires different enzymes and acid levels. The problem occurs when you mix foods that require many different enzyme and acid levels improperly. This leads to digestive problems and excessive mucus. Alternately, you get excessive amounts of gas, especially when you mix sugars that have high glycemic indexes (simple processed sugars like cake, and candy) with fatty proteins. Simple sugars usually do not combine well with protein. You know what they say about baked beans? Therefore, food combining becomes beneficial, since it is mandatory that these foods be digested and assimilated properly. Follow the rules below, and combine your foods accordingly.

Rule 1

Do not mix an array of foods, such as traditional dinners that combine salad, soup, entree, side dishes, and dessert. Although such dinners taste great, unless combined properly, which is highly unlikely, eating them dooms you to weight gain, bloat, allergies, digestive problems, fatigue, or all of the above. The explanation is simple: your digestive juices are regulated by the food you are eating. If you eat acidic foods, such as meats, grains, and dairy products, the chemical composition of your digestive enzymes is different from when you eat basic foods that are alkaline, such as fruits and vegetables. Mixing the wrong foods plays havoc with your enzyme and acid levels, preventing both kinds of food from being digested properly. The improperly digested foods now act as allergens, causing your body to secrete excess mucus to encapsulate the partially digested food (just like the body responds with any other allergen), leading to sinus and allergy conditions. Therefore, carbohydrates ferment rather than digest, and proteins tend to rot (decompose) instead of digest.

So, when eating, keep the types of foods in a meal down to a minimum, and use the recommendations below to help guide you. Below is a partial list of acidic and alkaline foods. More complete lists can be found on the Internet. Each meal should include a balance of acidic and alkaline foods to help regulate your body's pH. Before I discuss acidic and alkaline foods, let me first explain the meaning of pH.

The pH of Your Body

Before I discuss food combining, you must first understand the extreme importance food has on body chemistry through the pH scale. The pH scale (also known as the power of hydrogen) ranges from 0–14.

	<Acid					Water				Base>				
0	1	2	3	4	5	6	7	8	9	10	11	12	13	14

The scale is based on water as a neutral substance in the middle (seven). Anything below seven is considered acidic. The lower the number, the stronger the acid. For example, the acid in your stomach is between 1.0 and 3.5, and this acid is strong enough to eat through metal. Anything above seven is considered alkaline. The higher you go, the stronger the base, or alkali. The pH of your body's cells (one hundred trillion) is somewhere between 7.0 and 7.2, which is regulated by buffer systems in the body. Change this pH to 6.9 or 7.3 and you start to become biochemically imbalanced; if you go lower or higher, you will start the process of cellular degeneration, damage, and malfunction. If continued (left unchecked), death ensues rapidly.

As you can see, the pH balance is very delicate, and an imbalance can literally lead to death. The pH of your body is directly affected by what you eat, although we have buffer systems to help in this process. Through the right combination of foods, you can improve the pH of your body and alleviate undo stress on the buffer systems. Please see page 121 the acid/alkaline food charts. To make it simple, most fruits and vegetables, beans, and legumes are alkaline. Meat, fowl, fish, nuts/seeds, dairy, grains, and junk food are acidic. Remember, even if a food is acidic, there are foods with higher and lower acidity. The same holds true for alkaline foods.

Why are some foods considered acidic and some alkaline? You may even wonder how this is determined. Food is taken and burned until just the ash of the food is left. If the ash is alkaline, it means that there are many alkaline minerals present in the food. The higher the alkalinity, the higher the mineral content. If the ash of the food is acidic, it means that there are higher concentrations of amino acids (protein), fatty acids (fat), and acids from sugar (carbohydrate). The higher the amount of protein and fat, and the more complex the carbohydrate, the more acidic the food will be.

Alkaline and Acidic Food Charts

Alkaline-Forming Foods
(All fruits, vegetables, and rice)

Alfalfa	Almonds	Apples	Apricots
Artichokes	Avocados	Bananas (dried)	Bananas (ripe)
Beans, kidney	Beans, wax	Beans, string	Beets
Blackberries	Blueberries	Broccoli	Broth, vegetable
Butter	Cabbage	Cantaloupe	Carrots
Cauliflower	Celery	Cherries	Chicory
Coconuts	Coconut milk	Coffee substitute	Cranberries
Cucumbers	Currants	Dates	Endive
Eggplant	Figs	Garlic	Gelatin
Goat's milk	Grapefruit	Grapes	Honey
Huckleberries	Juices, fruit	Juices, vegetable	Kale
Kelp	Kohlrabi	Leek	Lettuce
Lemons	Limes	Loganberries	Meat substitutes
Mushrooms	Okra	Olives	Olive oil
Onions	Oranges	Parsley	Peaches
Pears	Pears, dried	Pears, fresh	Peppers, sweet
Peppermint leaves	Pineapple	Pineapple juice	Plums
Potatoes, sweet	Potatoes, white	Prunes	Pumpkins
Radishes	Raisins	Raspberries	Rice
Romaine	Rhubarb	Rutabagas	Soybeans
Soybean oil	Spinach	Sprouts	Squash
Strawberries	Swiss chard	Tomatoes	Turnips
Vegetable gelatin	Watercress	Watermelon	Wheat germ

Acid-Forming Foods
(Meats, dairy, and grains)

Barley	Beans, lima	Beans, white	Beef
Bread	Buttermilk	Cashew nuts	Cereals (read box)
Chestnuts	Chicken	Clams	Corn
Cornmeal	Cottage cheese	Crab	Crackers
Cream of Wheat	Duck	Eggs	Fish
Flour, white	Vital wheat gluten	Goose	Grape Nuts cereal
Ham	Lamb	Lentils	Lobster
Macaroni	Maize	Milk	Millet rye
Mutton	Oatmeal	Oysters	Peanuts
Peanut butter	Peas	Pecans	Pork chops
Rabbit	Rice, brown	Rice, polished	Rice, wild
Roquefort cheese	Rye flour	Sauerkraut	Spaghetti
Turkey	Veal chops	Vinegar	Walnuts

Page 110

Properly Combining Foods

Follow the examples below, which show you how to combine your foods properly:

Always combine an acid with an alkaline food.

1. For example, when eating protein that is high in fat (acid), use vegetables (alkaline) as your first choice, since they have fewer calories in large portions. Fatty proteins, such as red meat and dairy mix well with vegetables, creating the proper acid-alkaline balance for excellent digestion. Different proteins and vegetables impact people differently, so write down how you feel after the meal and over the next twelve hours to find the perfect combination for you. Remember, you want to mix acids with alkaline foods to keep your pH as close to 7.2 as possible.

2. Do not mix large amounts of grains (pasta, breads, and cereals), which are acidic, with high-fat proteins (meat, cheese, and fowl), which are also acidic. An acid does not balance an acid well. Such is the case with cereal and milk, spaghetti and meatballs.

3. If you do mix proteins with your grains, eat small amounts and make sure you add vegetables and/or fruit to help create the acid-alkaline balance. Grains, cereals, pastas, pizza, breads, and rice could be eaten separately or combined with vegetables, such as a small salad or vegetable portion.

4. Eat fruits/juices (alkaline) separately or as a small meal or snack. Small amounts of dairy (yogurt,

cream) or nuts and seeds could accompany the meal, since they are acidic.

5. A word of caution for people who prefer to be vegan. Eating mostly fruits, vegetables, and beans will increase your alkalinity. Remember, being too alkaline is just as bad as being too acidic. Make sure you have sufficient acid in your system to balance this alkalinity.

6. Diet soda, carbonated drinks, beer, and hard liquor are not to be used as a beverage with your meals. Instead, drink water, coffee/tea, wine, or milk. Whatever you drink, make sure you sip as opposed to swallow. You do not want to dilute acids and digestive juices from doing their jobs.

7. Always sip water with your meals, since it has a neutral pH and can help balance your acid/alkaline ratio, acting as a buffer between acidic and alkaline foods. For example, if your meal was too acidic, then water (which is neutral) can have an alkalizing effect on your meal. On the other hand, if your meal was too alkaline, water can have an acidic effect on your meal. So guess what? Drink water all day long; it balances your body's pH.

8. Based on our heritage, some of us require a slightly higher percentage of acid-forming or alkaline foods. For example, if you crave red meat, eggs, or cheese, which are extremely acidic, and come from a German heritage, then your diet will lean toward the acidic side. On the other hand, if you

crave vegetables or fruits, which are alkaline, and fish and rice, which are less acidic than red meats, then your diet would lean toward the alkaline side of this list. We should aim for ratios of 50–50 (acid/alkaline) to 60–40 (either way).
Please note that climate and physical stress can alter the above percentages.

If you now suffer from any of the following conditions, they may be the result of improper food combining: digestive complaints, sinus conditions, allergic reactions, fatigue, hyperactivity, headaches, or arthritic conditions.

When you eat meals that are extremely acidic or alkaline on a continuous basis, you will develop many health problems. This is due to stressing the buffer systems in the body and shifting your pH higher or lower than 7.0–7.2. Long-term, this can lead to cellular malfunction, damage, and death. A blood chemistry test can help determine whether you require more acid than alkaline and which proteins and carbohydrates are best for you. If you follow the above guidelines, you will notice that your digestion will improve, along with your overall health.

For more information about this very powerful blood test, you can contact my office directly at 561-627-3810 or e-mail me at drcima@cimahealth.com

18

Food Preparation

It is not only necessary to eat quality foods, but these foods need to be prepared so that they remain nourishing. Follow these guidelines when you prepare your foods. Broil, bake, barbecue, steam, stir-fry, toast, and fry with a light vegetable oil or butter. Use herbs, spices, and sea salt to enhance the flavoring and add natural healing elements. Keep food preparation to a minimum, and remember to keep it simple.

Number of Meals during the Day

Eat anywhere from a minimum of four to six meals per day. Decide when you want to eat, and eat at those times. You know when you are hungry and when you are not, so eat just before you are starving, and this will curb your appetite. Your meals do not have to be large; they could consist of one to two pieces of fruit and some nuts, for example. Meals should range from a few hundred calories to not more than a thousand calories. Take your time when eating, and relax after your meals. Relaxing after a meal helps you further digestion and reduce the risk of indigestion. Chew your foods slowly so they can be digested properly in the mouth, which will set the stage for the rest of digestion. As mentioned before, drink (sip) water with most of your meals, and if you drink alcohol, drink before your meal and very little with the meal. This allows the digestive juices to remain concentrated and do a more effective job with digestion. Take any supplementation at the beginning or just before meals. Supplements mixed with food during digestion assimilate much faster than when taken alone.

Between Meals

Always fill out your diet diaries. This habit will create your blueprint for your success. Points to follow when filling out your diet diary:

- ❖ Always write down what you eat and drink.
- ❖ Make sure you keep track of your protein, fat, carbohydrate, and caloric intake.
- ❖ List any supplements you are taking.
- ❖ Note how you feel and look.
- ❖ Write down your weight as well as your body composition, if you know it.
- ❖ Write out your exercise program for the day.

What We Have Accomplished So Far

So far, from a dietary standpoint, I have shown you rules to:

- ❖ Clean up your diet.
- ❖ Pick foods that you love to eat.
- ❖ Create the proper caloric intake.

- ❖ Create the proper protein, fat, and carbohydrate intake.
- ❖ Create the proper food combinations.
- ❖ Create the ideal preparation and ambience.

If you can live within these guidelines most of the time, you will create a well-balanced nutritional regime. The reality is that most of us find it hard to eat naturally, especially with the fast-paced lives that we lead. Sometimes fast food or no food is the only option. I agree it is difficult to prepare all of your meals and that you will slip up. That is OK if done in moderation and with the use of supplements to support your diet. Listen, if fast foods killed us as fast as some say they do, everyone would be dead. Faulty nutrition usually takes years, even decades of abuse to cause degeneration. Since we live in a fast-paced society with inferior-quality foods, supplements can give you the extra boost you do not get from the foods you eat. So exploring the use of supplements in our diet will be paramount if we are to survive in this hostile chemical environment. The next chapter explains a few reasons why supplements are a necessity in today's society.

19

Why the Need for Supplements?

I laugh when people or doctors say just eat right and you do not require supplements. Below are some reasons we need to supplement our diet in today's society:

❖ Today, foods are produced for quantity rather than quality. Even natural foods are deficient in vitamins and minerals due to the practice of overfarming land, which causes mineral and vitamin deficiencies. Therefore, although you may be getting vitamins and minerals, they are in insufficient amounts.

❖ Preservatives added to foods bind some of the available nutrients left in the food.

❖ Processing through extreme heating and freezing destroys the food molecules, causing the loss of vitamin and mineral content.

❖ The addition of a multitude of chemical oxidants and carcinogens, which have to be neutralized by the body's defense system, further depletes the body's vitamin and mineral reserve by taxing hormone and enzyme systems.

❖ People who smoke, drink, or take drugs require higher vitamin and mineral contents, due to the excessive oxidative and toxic effects of these vices.

❖ The effects of emotional stress cause an overutilization of hormones, which taxes the body's vitamin and mineral reserve.

❖ Physical activity, such as exercise or physical labor, increases the vitamin and mineral demands on your body.

❖ Environmental pollutants.

   ❖ According to the US Environmental Protection Agency: People exposed to toxic air pollutants at sufficient concentrations and durations may have an increased chance of getting cancer, damage to the immune system, as well as neurological, reproductive, respiratory, and other health problems.

   ❖ People are exposed to toxic air pollutants not only through the air they breathe but also through the effect of air pollutants on our soils and water. According to the Environmental Protection Agency, it is not uncommon for children to come into contact with polluted soil and then ingest these pollutants.

   ❖ According to the *World Book Encyclopedia*, more than 2.4 billion pounds of air pollution were expelled into the air in the United States in 1989. Conditions have only worsened.

   ❖ The *World Book Encyclopedia* also cited a study that found 188 million pounds of chemicals were discharged into our lakes, streams, and rivers, and one billion pounds of chemicals were released into the ground, threatening our natural groundwater sources.

❖ Many recent studies have found that our water contains traces of Prozac, Zoloft, estrogen, and numerous other pharmaceuticals, because our sewage treatment centers cannot eliminate them, writes Dr. Don Colbert MD in his book "What You Don't Know May Be Killing You".

If that doesn't shock you, maybe this will. A study by the Environmental Working Group found how much pollution enters our bodies by checking blood in the placentas of newborn children:

Until this study was done, it was assumed by scientists that the unborn child was protected from toxic chemicals. This study tested blood from ten newborn infants for a range of chemical pollutants, many of which are associated with abnormal development and poor health. On average, the infants were tested for over 280 different industrial chemicals in their blood. They found:

❖ 180 chemicals that cause cancer in humans.
❖ 217 chemicals that are toxic to the brain and nervous system.
❖ 208 chemicals that cause birth defects.

So, if an unborn baby cannot get away from these pollutants, then what chance do we stand? A plethora of toxic waste 150,000 strong are found in the air you breathe,

the water you drink, and the soil where we grow our food. These chemicals continue to traumatize and overtax hormone and enzyme systems necessary to neutralize, encapsulate, destroy, and remove these nasty carcinogens from our bodies.

The need for additional vitamin and nutritional support is an absolute necessity in today's environment. The right vitamin and mineral support is like having money in the bank and is necessary to ensure excellent health. If we need supplementation, we must know what and how much we need. We also want the best quality of supplementation we can get our hands on, pharmaceutical grade, or what we call neutraceutical grade.

First let me state that supplements are used to supplement your diet; they are not used in place of it. Do not use a supplement as a replacement for a proper diet.

Supplements: The Different Groups

In order to develop the right supplemental regime for your program, you must understand how each supplemental formulation works. Today, supplements are high-tech, and because of this, we have a better chance surviving our polluted universe and its adverse effects on our health. Supplements are necessary in today's society. Maybe you could have gotten away with not taking supplements in the past, but you won't be able to indefinitely. If you think you can, good luck! I will show you how to put together a broad spectrum formulation as well as a focused one. Let us first look at the various groups of supplements and offer a brief overview of what they do and how to choose supplements that are what I call bioavailable.

Bioavailability refers to the body's ability to use this supplement. For example, the raw material used to produce the supplement could have been made synthetically. Synthetic vitamins are a mirror image of what the real vitamin looks like. Therefore, it acts differently than the real one. It would be like putting a right-handed glove on your left hand; it would not fit properly and would limit your dexterity. On the other hand, just as food processing damages food, the supplemental formulation process can damage the vitamin, mineral, tissue concentrate, homeopathic remedy, etc. in that supplement. Therefore, the quality of the processing is just as important as the raw materials that are used to make the supplement.

Below is a classification of the different supplements that are used. Treat them like gold, for they are far more precious. Each particular supplement provides a specific use for the body:

- ❖ Vitamins
- ❖ Minerals
- ❖ Cellular tissue concentrates
- ❖ Herbs
- ❖ Homeopathic remedies

At the end of this section, are four formulations that have proven beneficial to myself, my family, and my patients as a dietary support or in the treatment of many of their health conditions. I highly recommend that you use these supplements, because they are pure, natural, and potent. Remember: Vitamins, minerals, and cellular tissue concentrates are used as food supplements for continued growth and repair of body cells, whereas herbal and homeopathic remedies are used as medicines to treat symptoms or diseases.

Vitamins

Vitamin deficiencies have long been known to cause all kinds of health conditions. The general function or purpose of vitamins is to act as coenzymes (help enzymes function) and to affect the pH of membranes. This is a fancy way of saying that vitamins affect the movement of food and oxygen entering the cell as well as the movement of cell waste and carbon dioxide leaving the cell. Vitamins are divided into two groups: water-soluble and fat-soluble.

Water-soluble vitamins (they dissolve in water):

Water-soluble vitamins are further broken down into acid and alkaline groups. For example, Vitamin C and certain B vitamins, such as pantothenic acid and para-aminobenzoic acid, are in the acidic group. Please note that acidic vitamins acidify membranes, making them more permeable (things can pass in and out of cells more freely). This is why vitamin C is good for colds, since it makes the membrane more permeable, so the cells can discharge the toxic metabolic wastes faster. Thiamin, riboflavin, choline, and inositol are in the alkaline group. Alkaline B vitamins make membranes less permeable. Therefore, the proper balance of acid and alkaline vitamins is necessary to maintain membrane pH and function.

Fat-soluble vitamins (they dissolve in fat):

Fat-soluble vitamins are vitamins D, E, K, and A. Guess where you find fat-soluble vitamins? In fats! This is why fat is important. It contains fat-soluble vitamins that are necessary for life. When fats are processed, the fat-soluble vitamins are removed by the processing. Some people crave fat because they are not meeting their fat-soluble vitamin intake. Therefore, they continue to crave fat. If you give such people the right fatty proteins, which contain fat-soluble vitamins, it will decrease their craving for fat. The purpose of fat-soluble vitamins is to produce hormones, enzymes, and antibodies and coat the cell membranes, preventing damage to the membrane from the oxidative effects of oxygen. Oxygen will dry out the membrane surface, causing problems with cellular exchange. By increasing these fat-soluble vitamins, you can protect and maintain membrane permeability, which is essential for cellular exchange.

The general function of all vitamins is to maintain and regulate all cell membrane activity. This ensures that substances, such as food, can pass through membranes when they enter the cell and that cell waste products can leave the cell. So, an excellent vitamin supplement will help you maintain health in a fast-paced society. When you choose your vitamin supplements, please do not use vitamins that are synthetically made; contain fillers, coloring, or additives; and do not have a high enough dosage to ensure that you can maintain your recommended daily allowance. Don't be a Scrooge when purchasing your supplements—remember, you get what you pay for.

At the end of this section, I have included a list of the best vitamin and mineral complexes that my family, my patients, and I use.

Minerals

The purpose of a mineral is to transport substances through the body. Minerals act as magnets and polarize (pull) chemicals (hormones, enzymes, and antibodies) from one area of the body to another. Certain minerals have an affinity for specific glands and are stored in these specific glands and organs. Such is the case with iodine in the thyroid, iron and copper in the liver, and chromium and zinc in the pancreas for insulin regulation.

In order for minerals to be used by the body, they must be in the ionized state. In other words, the mineral must have a positive or negative charge (because they act like magnets). Minerals that are inert (no charge) have a toxic effect on the body. I mention this because the type of supplement that you purchase must contain minerals that can ionize easily. The following will help you to choose a mineral supplement that is bioavailable and easily ionized.

Chelated minerals:

These minerals are attached to a protein. This allows for better mineral absorption and digestion by the body, as opposed to a supplement that only contains the mineral. The reason is that minerals are attached to proteins in nature. You normally do not eat pure minerals. Chelated minerals are an ideal combination with specific tissues, which will be discussed next.

Colloidal minerals (minerals in suspension):

These minerals are highly bioavailable. These minerals are in suspension and are readily available for body use.

Ionic minerals:

It's rather obvious that if we could get minerals in an ionized state would be ideal. Well, not only can we get minerals in an ionized state, we can also receive all the necessary minerals for body function. It is the perfect mineral supplement/condiment, and it is called sea salt.

Sea Salt

Mother Nature's perfect condiment and mineral formulation is sea salt. People have been misinformed when it comes to sea salt; they confuse it with table (white) salt. Sea salt is a healthy and necessary condiment in anyone's diet for the following reasons. The first reason is that it contains all of the sixty-six or so minerals that the human body needs to function. Sea salt also contains all of the micro-minerals, such as silicon and boron, which are deficient in today's diets due to mineral-deficient soil. Table salt, due to processing, removes the majority of these micro-minerals except for sodium and chloride. Therefore, you receive little if any micro-mineral benefit.

The minerals in sea salt are in the same proportion to the minerals found in your blood. In other words, these minerals are readily absorbed due to the balanced mineral relationship with our blood. In fact, when blood or plasma is not available in hospitals, saline (salt) solution is used in place of the blood or plasma.

The minerals in sea salt are also in an ionized state. As mentioned above, the body can only use minerals that are in an ionized state (that have a positive or negative charge). If the minerals are not in an ionized state (inert, no charge), the body cannot use the mineral. For example, have you ever put table salt in water (to gargle perhaps) and watched it dissolve (ionize) before you drank it? After dissolving, the salt starts to reappear on the bottom of the glass. This occurs as the table salt returns to an inert state. What happened was the sodium and chloride molecule split apart into a sodium and chloride ion, which the body can now use. Due to the high concentration of sodium and chloride, the sodium and chloride had a greater chance to reassociate (attach) and settled on the bottom of the glass in an inert form. This is what causes you to retain water and leads to heart and kidney problems. This is not the case with sea salt, which ionizes easily and tends to stay that way, due to the multitude of minerals repelling and attracting continually. Next time you go to the beach, let me know how much salt you find on the sand.

Sea salt brings out food flavor, enhancing your taste buds, as it improves body function. It tastes great, and at the same time, you are supplementing your meals with a perfectly balanced mineral formulation made by Mother Nature/God. Bon Appétit! To purchase the finest sea salt on the market at the best price, please check out the end of this section.

Cell/Tissue Concentrates

Cellular tissue therapy aka glandular therapy dates back to 1400 BC. The premise of cellular tissue therapy is to use a healthy gland or organ "tissue concentrate" in pill, spray or liquid form to repair a damaged gland or organ. This premise makes sense when you analyze the following:

❖ Each gland or organ is made from different types of proteins.
❖ The type of protein dictates what the organ looks like, as well as how it functions.

This is why your liver not only looks different from your heart—it works differently as well. What makes one protein different from another is its amino acid combination. Proteins are made up of units called amino acids. There are twenty-one different amino acids that can attach and create chains, thousands of amino acids long, thus making up 150,000 different proteins that create the human body. Change one amino acid in a chain and you have a different protein, with different properties and characteristics. This is why there are no two people who look alike, unless they are identical twins and even they are not totally identical. The possible number of combinations of amino acids to form different types of proteins is astronomical.

If we could ingest a protein as a food source that resembled the amino acid structure of that organ, then you would have a greater chance of that organ getting the proper amino acids in the proper balance (similar to the effects of sea salt, with its proportionate relationship to blood). Therefore, by ingesting thyroid, liver, heart, stomach, and pancreas in a tissue concentrate, you help the body by giving it the identical raw materials that it needs to repair and rebuild those particular glands and organs.

What enhances cellular tissue therapy is having the right mineral chelated to the right cell and tissue. So, not only is the organ receiving the needed amino acids but the minerals as well. This, coupled with the specific vitamin support (for example fat-soluble vitamins for the liver) for that particular gland or organ, makes for a wonderful support package. So, cellular tissue therapy is utilized to support a specific gland or organ from a nutritional standpoint.

Cell tissue concentrates along with vitamins and minerals are the only supplements that repair, rebuild, and provide cells with raw materials and genetic material to create new cells. For the past thirty-five years, I have used tissue concentrates to treat my own health and that of my family and patients. I have seen many conditions—including diabetes, heart and respiratory conditions, hormonal imbalances, and digestive complaints—resolved through the use of cellular tissue concentrates. These cellular tissue concentrates are made from the finest raw materials, and the processing is second to none, making these the finest neutraceutical grade cellular tissue concentrates on the market today.

Herbal Remedies

Herbs come from various parts of plants or other vegetation. The roots, bark, flowers, leaves, buds, or resin (sap) can be used to make pills, teas, oils/creams, and condiments. The medicinal properties of herbs have been known and used for centuries by the Chinese. Herbs really are one of God's natural remedies. Herbal formulas are utilized by the body to promote healing and symptomatic relief without the severe adverse side effects of most medications. Herbal formulas are very powerful and can have a dramatic effect on the body. I do not recommend that you take any herbal formula without the direction of a qualified physician. Herbs, for the most part are natural medications that heal the body, unlike vitamins, minerals, and glandulars, which are continually needed by the body for growth and repair. Herbal formulations are used when there is a health condition or problem. Herbal remedies are given based on a symptomatic diagnosis by the physician until the patient is well. At that point, the herbal formula is usually discontinued, unless otherwise indicated. Constantly and continually taking herbs is not recommended unless under the directions of someone who is qualified in this field.

Homeopathy

Homeopathy was founded and developed by German-born Dr. Samuel Hahnemann in the early nineteenth century. The basic premise of homeopathy is that you treat like with like, using very diluted dosages. During the nineteenth century, malaria and scarlet fever were what cancer and heart disease are today: deadly killers. The cure for malaria was quinine, and the cure for scarlet fever was belladonna. What Dr. Hahnemann found interesting was that in healthy individuals, quinine caused the symptoms of malaria, and belladonna caused the symptoms of scarlet fever. Dr. Hahnemann concluded, hypothetically, that this might be true for many other diseases, and he spent the majority of his research noting the symptomatic response any chemical, metal, or substance had on the human body. When Dr. Hahnemann found a substance that mimicked the symptoms of a particular disease, he used that chemical in a diluted form to treat that disease.

For example, a 1X solution of any homeopathic remedy is equal to one drop of that remedy in fourteen gallons of water. You have dilutions up to 100X, which creates an energetic molecular effect on the body. In other words, the body reads the molecular imprint of the remedy and then reacts, based on what it reads. A crude example of this is when you get a flu shot. In the shot, there is a weakened strain of the virus that causes the disease you're trying to prevent from infecting the body. Because of the viruses diluted, weakened state, your body's defense systems have time to rally to the occasion. This leads to a buildup of antibodies specific to that virus, and now your defense system is beefed up, ready for an all-out assault on that strain of virus.

Homeopathy works on the same principle. Give the body a tickle dosage, and it will stimulate the body's defense and endocrine systems into action, as if World War III was about to start. Homeopathic remedies may include tinctures of vitamins, minerals, herbs, glandulars, and minerals. They are also made from diseased tissue, microorganisms (such as bacteria virus, fungi), environmental pollutants, and radiation. These particular remedies detoxify, vaccinate, and purge the body of harmful chemicals, toxic agents, bacteria, and viruses.

Homeopathic remedies are typically used when you are experiencing a health condition. Typically, you visit a qualified physician and receive a diagnosis along with a homeopathic remedy. When the condition clears, the remedy is discontinued, unlike vitamins, minerals, and glandulars, which are used as building blocks to repair and rebuild the body. Homeopathic remedies, just like herbs, are used to combat a specific illness or condition and then discontinued when the symptomatic complaints stop.

20

Creating Your Supplemental Profile

When I ask my patients if they take supplements, they usually say yes. When I ask them what they take and why they take it, the confusion really starts. Most people take supplements based on what somebody told them or what they saw in a magazine, on the Internet, or TV. Half the time what they are taking is based on erroneous information, and in reality they do not even need to take the supplement, which means they are just taking supplements and wasting money. In fact, I'm willing to bet you that most of the supplements people take are not even digested and utilized by the body and are excreted as waste. So how do you know what supplements to take, why you should take them, and in what amounts?

At the beginning of this book I stated that I would give you 20 percent of the information that will give you 80 percent of your result. In this case, it will be more like 95 percent. When taking supplementation, I use a very simple but effective program that gives me everything I need. Remember, supplementation is used to supplement your diet and does not take the place of wholesome foods. Let's create a general nutritional support program that will give you everything that you need.

We already explained the need for vitamins, minerals, and phytonutrients (essential nutrients from plants) that our bodies require daily.

So let's get supplements that:

- ❖ Come from natural raw materials that are highly bioavailable with a simple delivery system.
- ❖ Processing does not damage or destroy or chemically alter the vitamins, minerals, RNA, DNA, etc. that are in the natural raw material.

  This constitutes a true neutraceutical: the highest quality, concentration, and perfection of the raw material.

So over the last four decades I've come up with the perfect supplementation program that I utilize daily. It's a basic program that everyone can utilize and gives you a near perfect blend of every vitamin, mineral, micro-mineral, cellular tissue concentrate and phytonutrient that you would probably ever need.

I call it the balanced nutritional protocol.

BALANCED NUTRITIONAL PROTOCOL

Below are four products that will give you just about all the general support you would require.

1. Cimasystem multivitamin/mineral formulation 1

2. Cimasystem Active cellular therapy formulation 2

3. Sea salt: microminerals

4. Nanno greens Phytonutrients from fifty plus plants, fruits and herbs

   For a cost of around seventy dollars per month, you can have a complete supplementation program that will give you everything you require:
   I know most people who purchase supplements pay much more for a poorer grade supplement. Those of you that take some generic supplement, you are still paying too much for so little. *Excellent health does not cost—it pays.*
   To order, and save 10 percent please call 561-627-3810, or order from my website www. cimahealthandwellness.com.

Now I know some of you might want to get more specific and talk about this specific nutrient and that specific nutrient for this particular reason or health condition. I will now address that. There are many people out there right now that are looking for supplements to help them heal their health problems. So when some guru tells them to take this particular supplement for this health problem, they think it will work. If it were that easy to determine biochemical malfunction in the body, I wasted a lot of decades studying nutrition, biochemistry, cellular physiology, endocrinology, and laboratory diagnosis. I could have just taken out my "Cookbook Nutritional Manual" and looked up digestive problems to find the right recipe. How ridiculousness does that sound? I decided to take the high road and really put my nose to the grindstone, because I knew my patients' health was in jeopardy. I was looking for a way to truly diagnose biochemical malfunction in the body. Below is the most accurate scientific method that I know of to assess not only what supplementation you would need as an individual for your particular health problems but what type of diet will best support your health.

Back in the late 1970s, I was introduced to a way to analyze a patient's nutritional deficiencies. At that time, I was looking for ways to objectively evaluate and examine a patient from a valid chemical viewpoint. I felt that I would need to know two things about the patient in order to determine a proper nutritional program.

❖ What are the right foods for each individual? As clichés tell us, "One man's food is another man's poison" and "You are what you eat." Just like we are all physically different, we are all biochemically different to some degree. This would be synonymous with putting the right fuel into your automobile.

❖ You also a product of what you digest, assimilate, and metabolize. You might eat the greatest of food but because you can't digest, assimilate, or metabolize the foods, you do not get much nutritional benefit from them. This is synonymous with a car that needs a tune-up.

Then, I found the perfect test, a test that all physicians would say was reliable and valid—a blood chemistry test. It's called a SMAC 25 CBC/Diff, which is a general scanning test that all doctors use. It gives the doctor a general idea of how the body is functioning chemically. This test, when examined correctly, can also tell you nutritional deficiencies in your diet as well as what glands and organs may need supplemental support to prevent organ and glandular degeneration. The test will help you to identify health problems before they get to that life-threatening state.

So if you're going to spend money on supplements, at least spend money on supplements that are going to help improve your health. Do not guess about it.

I recommend this test to anyone, especially if you have a health condition caused by a biochemical imbalance. If you are over thirty, you probably already have a biochemical imbalance.

This test will identify problem areas as well as determine your nutritional profile, giving you the best starting baseline. This is about as specific and focused as you can get using nutritional support. For more information on this blood chemistry analysis, you can call my office 561-627-3810 or e-mail me at drcima@cimahealth.com. You can also visit my website www.cimahealthandwellness.com.

Section Four:

Let Your Presence Command Attention: The Physical Side

Pain Sucks

Our physical body is very important for our survival. After all, we need a functional body to perform work. We need a body free of pain to be efficient and effective at performing whatever tasks our mind wants us to perform. Like a race car, your body has to perform at optimum levels in order to reach the winner's circle.

Due to physical stress exerted on the body through the effects of gravity, your body has undergone some serious damage. Physical stresses such as falls, accidents, sports injuries, obesity, occupational hazards, and lack of exercise have all contributed to this physical trauma.

Besides wanting a functional body, we also look at the physical body as a thing of beauty. The very first thing you notice about anyone is his or her physical appearance. Did you know that physical appearance counts more than anything else on a job interview? There is something intriguing, mesmerizing, and exciting about the human body. That is why we all want a beautiful body and why many people will go to any length to achieve one. But few ever do. It is easier to become a billionaire than to develop a beautiful and healthy body. Oh, sure, when you're between twenty and thirty it's easy, but not when you're forty, fifty, sixty, or seventy.

Pain Sucks.

Pain sucks! I lived with it; I treat it; and I've watched people's lives destroyed because of it. According to Dr. Mehmet Oz, "Pain is the number one reason patients go to the doctor." While we've all experienced some form of physical pain in our lives, our injuries are usually short-lived. For about 35 percent of Americans, however, pain escalates into a chronic problem lasting three to six months, or even longer.

Chronic pain affects 30-50 million Americans and social and productivity costs of $100 billion annually. This comes from the Joint Commission on Accreditation Of Healthcare Organizations.

Pain may not kill you, but you may wish that you were dead. It interferes with life and your ability to function. You cannot do things as far as your occupation goes; your sports activities are curtailed, as are the simple activities of daily living. You find going to the john a chore in itself. There is no way you can be in chronic, unrelenting pain and be in a positive emotional state. In fact, it is impossible, because pain in itself is a negative emotional state. Even if you take pain medication, the cause is still present, and the pain is still there to some degree.

So, first and foremost, conditioning the human body to counteract the cause of physical pain will be completely discussed in this section. I also bring your attention to the part of this section that deals with the treatment of the cause of this pain. Trust me—these problems get worse, not better. Thinking they'll improve will only bring more suffering, pain, and disability.

Please do not take your pain lightly even if you can live with it. So many patients say they can until the day they can no longer do it, and surgery is their only option. The problem with surgeries is they are also ineffective for the most part. They don't get to the cause of the problem and require follow-up surgeries, causing more pain and suffering until the only thing left may be suicide. Pain destroys your will to live and your emotional state. Chronic pain makes life a living nightmare.

21

Beauty and Grace

When we blend the function of the physical body with its beauty (physical aesthetics), we get beauty and grace. This is why we experience awe when we watch a professional gymnast, quarterback, baseball player, basketball player, golfer, skier, surfer, or the Miss America Pageant.

When we see the one person with the greatest physical development in a particular sport coupled with a functioning graceful body, that person's beauty and grace mesmerize us. Not only is physical fitness necessary for our survival but it has a dramatic effect on our mental attitude. I am sure that all people would love to have a beautiful body that is physically effective and efficient. Can you imagine the exhilaration you would feel if your body could perform at a professional level in your favorite sport? Stop and think for a moment. If your body were able to perform this way, how dramatically would it affect your life? Some of you might be excited if you could walk a few blocks at a moderate pace, but just imagine if your body had very few physical limitations. Think about how much better and easier your life would be. You would have tremendous amounts of energy and physical strength, much more than you need to go through life. Your physical capacity should be ten times more than you really need it to be. When you possess these qualities, it is like having money in the bank.

So, now that you have a better understanding of how important your body is to your life, let's analyze how you can create the necessary changes in your physical frame. Let us first realize that caring for your body is an ongoing process, and the more mature you become, the more work you need. I love to use the analogy of the automobile when discussing the body, since it is very appropriate. If you were to purchase the car of your dreams, what car would it be? Would it be a high-performance, luxury/deluxe model or a sturdy work vehicle?

The type of vehicle you choose is determined by your needs. If performance is what you're after, then that is what you would look for in a vehicle. Obviously, you would want a body that would last a long time, a body sturdy enough to handle any physical demands placed on it without breaking down (aches and pains) and with all the creature comforts of a luxury car (beauty and grace). Of course, you would choose a body style (physique) that would fit not only your functional needs but your aesthetic needs as well. I really do not care how old you are; you can still condition your body.

Just as collectors restore classic automobiles, you can restore your body. Just as there are body and fender shops that fix your car after it's damaged in an accident, there are body and fender shops for your body. So, start to think about what you want your body to do and what you want it to look like. Using the principles set forth in this book, you will create the body you have always wanted but have not yet been able to achieve.

22

How the Body Functions

If you are going to improve something, you need to know how it works, what makes it tick. Let me ask you a simple question: how does your body function? If you cannot answer this simple question, you do not stand a chance of making significant improvements. To create a clear understanding of body function, I will at times make connections between the body and machines. After all, machinery is a man-made copy of the organs and glands that the human body needs to function. By using the design of the human body as a template, most scientists/ inventors invent or create useful machines. Such is the case with engines, computers, electrical appliances, etc. Our bodies run on electricity just as a light bulb does, pure and simple. I could jazz it up and state that your body runs on a biochemical, electromagnetic phenomenon, which is under the control of the neuroendocrine axis, but I won't.

When you understand what I am about to explain, it will change your life forever. Your body is composed of one hundred trillion cells, which is roughly fifteen thousands times the population of earth and is under the control of your nervous system. The nervous system acts as a communication line linking all one hundred trillion cells. Your nervous system is like AT&T service or the Internet. In fact, the purpose of the nervous system is to coordinate and control the function of every cell, tissue, gland, and organ in the body. Can you imagine a population that is fifteen thousand times our population where everyone is working together in perfect harmony? In fact, the first system to develop in the human embryo is the nervous system, known as the primitive streak. This premature nervous system guides and directs the various cells into their respective positions (much like a blueprint), creating a fully formed human being in nine months.

Your nervous system is linked to every system, organ, gland, and tissue in the body. It controls the function of all these tissues, including your heart, stomach, lungs, kidneys, spleen, and reproductive organs. It also sends and receives messages from the brain, coordinating your hundred trillion cells so that your heart, stomach, lungs, kidneys, spleen, and reproductive organs remain healthy. If you affect this communication between the brain and a body part, you affect the performance of that gland or organ. When you affect this communication, you are literally affecting the nerve supply to that body part.

The number of neurological impulses per second determines the language of how your body communicates with itself. Like a Morse code of neurological impulses, the brain directs and communicates through the nervous system what the body should do each millisecond that you are alive. Can you imagine maintaining the needs of a hundred trillion people each day, so that all could live in perfect harmony? The thought of coordinating and communicating with that many people, getting them to do what is needed, is incomprehensible, especially considering how hard it is to get a family of six to agree on where to go for dinner.

People do not comprehend how amazing their body truly is. There is no way that we even come close to duplicating what the body is capable of doing. We can create simplistic imitations, such as computers and machinery, which we marvel at, since man built them. The human body created by God is OK, we seem to think, but it is not as fancy as my new ten-billion-gigabyte computer with the front axial drive. Your brain makes the most sophisticated computer look like a Mickey Mouse toy.

So your brain, spinal cord and the rest of your nervous system control, coordinate, and organize all of the functions between the cells, tissues, organs, glands so that all work in perfect harmony when in a state of health.

So what would cause my nervous system to malfunction?

Causes of Neurologic Malfunction

There are three factors that cause your nervous system to malfunction, interfering with the intelligence that controls body function and health:

1. Chemical stresses, such as diet and environmental pollutants.
2. Physical stresses, such as falls and accidents.
3. Mental stresses, such as finances, family, and work.

Do these sound familiar? If these three factors affect the nervous system, you must learn how to reduce the effects of all three. In this section I will discuss how you can reduce physical stress on the nervous system.

The Protectors and Supporters of Our Nervous System

Our nervous system is so fragile that it is protected by bone. The skull and spinal column encase and protect our brain and spinal cord from serious injury. When trauma or physical injury is greater than the bone strength, as when fractures occur, paralysis, brain damage, or death can result.

Your muscles, tendons, and ligaments support, protect, and move the bones. The nerves contract the muscles, which then move the bones. Therefore:

❖ Bones protect the nerves,
❖ Muscles and the other soft tissues (ligaments, tendons) support and move the bones, through proper nerve supply.
❖ Nerves, muscles, and bones share a commonality, whereby one has a dramatic effect on the other. If you physically damage muscle, you affect the movement of bones affecting ligaments, and damage/irritate nerves, causing pain (Next Page).

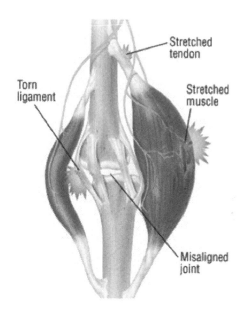

Torn
ligament

Stretched
tendon

Stretched
muscle

Misaligned
joint

This is why it is imperative to strengthen your musculo-skeletal system to overcome the effects that gravity has on your body. I know you cannot really feel gravity until you challenge the laws of gravity (such as stepping off a ten-story building), but gravity is constantly forcing your body into the ground. That is why when people reach their sixties, seventies, and eighties, they often cannot walk. It is the result of seventy-five years of gravitational effects on the body. Notice the infliction and crippling effect gravity has on our elderly population. Wheelchairs, walkers, canes, and severe unrelenting pain are what you have to look forward to. Isn't that nice?

Do you know how these terrible problems start? Well, they usually start in childhood or the teen years as a minor back or neck complaint from a sports injury, fall, or accident. They're not painful enough to send you to the doctor, but they're painful enough to get your attention. As months turn into years, the pains grow worse, and as years turn into decades, damage and degeneration may require surgery, fusion, or joint replacement.

By this time, your fate is sealed, and your future is not very bright. Not only is your movement affected, but your nervous system is now compromised by this lack of support and protection. The bone degeneration and damaged soft tissues (muscles, ligaments, tendons, and cartilage) act in a detrimental fashion and impede nerve supply. Instead of supporting and protecting the nerves, they irritate, traumatize, and damage them, setting up a host of complaints. This nerve irritation not only affects muscles but also affects the function of organs and glands that are controlled by those nerves. For example, injuries causing low back pain may also cause problems with your kidneys, bladder, large intestine, and sex organs.

So, care of the human frame or physical body is important not only for movement and support, but for proper nerve function as well, which is our major concern when dealing with our health. If you want to live for 150 years, you do not want to be confined to a wheelchair, nor do you want to be hobbling around in severe pain. You want to be out participating in the sport of your choice—running, swimming, swinging, throwing, kicking, or whatever you like—at age 120. What fun would life be if you could not walk and were in constant pain all the time?

By the way, the bones, muscles, and other soft tissues support, protect, and hold your organs and glands in place as well. Let's think of a skyscraper to illustrate this point. When building a skyscraper, first you see the steel girders that make up the frame of the building. This is analogous to your skeletal system (your bones). Then builders pour the concrete floors and attach the exterior walls to this main frame for support and protection. This is analogous to your muscles, ligaments, tendons, and cartilage. The electrical wiring is analogous to your nervous system. All of the appliances in the building, including the air-conditioning, heating, lighting, plumbing, etc. are analogous to your systems, organs, and glands. Note that if you have a sturdy building and foundation, you are secure in that building. However, if the foundation is weak, and the girders are rusted and bent, the housing authority condemns the building. If you were in a condemned building, you would not want to stay there, would you? You would want to move out. However, when you are talking about your body, you cannot move out, can you?

If you don't take care of your body, where else are you going to live?

Do you want to live in a shack or a palace? The choice is yours. Follow this section carefully, and I will show you how to transform your body into your palace, or your "temple," as the Bible says.

23

Conditioning the Human Frame (Body)

In order to condition the human body, you must use physical exercise, pure and simple. There are three classifications of exercise:

1. Stretching (flexibility)
2. Cardiovascular (aerobic)
3. Progressive resistance (anaerobic)

Each type of exercise will be discussed, including its necessity, guidelines to follow, and how to perform the exercise. But before we begin, I would like you to make some commitments to yourself. First, this is going to be a lifestyle change, which will require about three to five hours per week. Hey, you devote time to other important areas of your life, such as your job, family, or hobbies. Why not devote time to your health, since everything else depends on it? Without your health, you have no life. Besides, the three to five hours that you spend exercising will give you:

❖ Twice the energy.
❖ Twice the mental focus.

❖ Twice the physical power.

❖ The increased energy and power that you gain from exercise, not to mention the freedom from pain, could save you ten hours each week.

So, right now, pick three to five hours out of your busy week, and set them aside. This is your time, so if you wish to be alone to contemplate your thoughts, or if you prefer to exercise with friends, just do it. Secondly, I want you to develop your program using the right purpose. Your purpose will be your model or template that will forge the body of your dreams.

Your purpose should be as follows:

❖ I will create an exercise program that I love and look forward to.

❖ My program will create a healthy, functional, graceful body that I will consider a work of art.

Just like any other masterpiece, a healthy body represents a never-ending quest for perfection that I always strive to achieve. When you start to forge your dream body, you will be so excited and pumped up that you will dream, sleep, and think about exercise.

Exercise Will Become Your Escape into a New Reality— A New Beginning.

Exercise will be your mini-vacation every week; isn't that fun? When you're turning your body into a masterpiece, you have a never-ending list of goals to achieve. Once you reach a goal, you always have another to strive for. You are on a quest that becomes part of your existence, because your health is your existence. So, with your purpose established, have fun and stick to it. After a while, exercise will fit like a glove into your schedule, and when you get to that point, it is all downhill. Once you make these commitments to yourself, you are now ready to learn about exercise.

{ *Exercise does not consume time;*
it manufactures time. }

{ *Worth more than riches and fine gold,*
your body and health are things of beauty,
gifts from God that money cannot buy. }

24

The Philosophy, Science, and Art of Exercise

I want to create a brand-new viewpoint about exercise. If you view exercise as a philosophy, science, and art, then exercise becomes a little more intriguing. After all, I am not here to give you the same verbiage about exercise that you could pick up elsewhere but the essence of what exercise is all about. This will stimulate the way you think about your program. You will methodically build your program the way a builder constructs a mansion—systematically, detail by detail, every point taken into consideration. Therefore, the finished product is something to be proud of.

Exercise Is a Philosophy.
　　There are certain principles and truths about why and what you should do. Have you ever fallen into a pattern of exercise only to realize that, after a while, you stopped seeing much change? You may even have starved yourself, worked out countless hours, and still seen very little, if any, improvement for your trouble. That is because you did not know the philosophy or principles of exercise; for if you did, you could radically change how you look in no

time. There are many principles that you will have to follow in order to develop an effective and efficient program.

Exercise Is a Science.

You need to have some knowledge of exercise physiology (the study of how muscles and joints work and are stimulated) and anatomy (the study of muscle and joint location and motion). This knowledge helps back up the principles that you learn as well as determine the exercises you, as an individual, will need.

Exercise Is an Art.

You have to perform all exercises with perfect form. In other words, you are going to have to exercise the body a certain way in order to create the body you want, which will also be an art form. Not only is there artistic talent in performing the exercises using impeccable form, but your final product—your body—will be a work of art. So, let us first look at why we need to create a program using all three types of exercise, starting with stretching and flexibility training.

25

Stretching and Flexibility Training

In order to understand the importance of stretching and flexibility training, we must know something about joints, muscles, and movement. A simple joint is composed of two bones. The place where the bones join is called the joint. Between the bones, you have either cartilage or a disc (as in the spine) to act as a shock absorber between the bones. What holds your bones together are rubber-band-like structures called ligaments, and tendons attach muscle to bone. So tendons attach muscles to bones, and ligaments attach bones to bones. Nerve fibers then stimulate the muscle to contract, which pulls on the tendon, which moves the bone, which then moves the joint. See Fig.1.

FIG.1

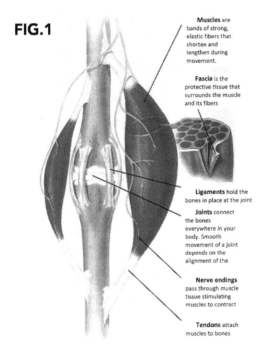

Muscles are bands of strong, elastic fibers that shorten and lengthen during movement.

Fascia is the protective tissue that surrounds the muscle and its fibers

Ligaments hold the bones in place at the joint

Joints connect the bones everywhere in your body. Smooth movement of a joint depends on the alignment of the

Nerve endings pass through muscle tissue stimulating muscles to contract

Tendons attach muscles to bones

This will now give you a better understanding of how each type of tissue functions in joint motion. Another interesting fact about muscle physiology is that muscles have an inborn (inherent) ability to contract. In medical circles, we say that a muscle maintains a certain level of tone (contraction) even when that muscle is in a relaxed state. This is why you need to stretch and increase flexibility, since muscle has this inborn tendency to contract.

Why Stretching and Flexibility Training Is So Important

As you go through life, at certain points you will encounter physical traumas to your body. I have been informed that the average infant hits its head two hundred times before it turns two years old. Some of you have been banging your heads a little longer. Therefore, throughout life, along with the effects of gravity, which no one can escape, we fall, get into accidents, develop sports injuries, and work in professions that create occupational hazards. Other things take their toll, such as being overweight or sitting/sleeping on uncomfortable furniture. Therefore, as you go through subsequent traumas, you traumatize the soft tissue (muscle, ligament, tendon, cartilage, and nerve), causing slight tears and fraying, particularly in the muscles, ligaments, and tendons. Fig. 2.

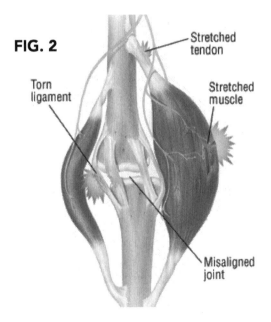

FIG. 2

Stretched tendon

Torn ligament

Stretched muscle

Misaligned joint

Muscles are also found in a state of spasm (increased tone), moving the joint out of alignment, which in turn irritates nerves, causing pain, weakness, and instability in the joint. This causes excessive wear and tear on the joint and leads to what doctors refer to as sprains, strains, tendonitis, bursitis, and capsulitis. If left uncorrected, the joint can undergo hard-tissue changes, such as arthritis, degeneration, and osteoporosis. Notice that arthritic or osteoporotic bones are misshapen. The joint becomes compressed due to wear and tear on cartilage and disc structures. Now the body tries to cement the injured joint together using calcium, which leads to an arthritic condition, followed by degenerative joint disease and then joint replacement. *If you want to reduce the risk of these problems, stretch and increase your flexibility!*

Now that you know why you should stretch and flexibility train, let me outline a program that will be safe and effective. Before starting any exercise regimen, I strongly recommend that you find a physician who can help you in this endeavor, especially if you have any health problems. Stretching daily helps create a routine (like brushing your teeth) that eventually becomes a habit. In fact, I look forward to stretching every morning, which I also use as "quiet time" to get in touch with my mind and body. By the way, the only way to gain flexibility is to stretch daily. When stretching and flexibility training, please follow the guidelines on the next page:

1. Stretch and flexibility train in the morning, evening, or both, depending on injuries or tight areas. Each session should last fifteen to thirty minutes.
2. Taking a hot shower before loosens the muscles.
3. Never perform ballistic or bouncing stretches that are painful. These exercises are dangerous and can cause a lot of joint damage.
4. Always use a comfortable, firm surface, and if there are low back or neck injuries, use a foam tube or rolled towel behind your neck and/or behind your knees.
5. Always start your stretching and flexibility training lying down and then proceed to sitting, kneeling, and standing.
6. Always spend more time on the tight muscles or tight side of the body.
7. Always use deep, relaxed breathing when stretching. When stretching a muscle, you must stretch and at the same time relax that muscle as far as you can comfortably. When you reach that point, you must focus on two things: breathing and blending your mind with that muscle (focus on relaxing it). Let me explain that last point further. When you reach the point in the stretch when the muscle starts to tighten and ache from the stretch, you now use breathing and mind/muscle relaxation to gain more stretch in that muscle or joint by relaxing it. This is what I mean by stretch and flexibility training, you relax and elongate (stretch) the muscle at the same time. When you reach that point, focus on deep, relaxed breathing, gaining

a little more length with each exhalation. In other words, as you exhale, you will be able to push the stretch a little more and then hold that position while you inhale relaxing that muscle. Then, when you exhale, you may gain a little more, or hold that position longer. Then repeat the cycle one more time. By this point, you can hold that position for another ten or fifteen seconds. Then release the stretch slowly. During this time, your mental focus should be on consciously relaxing that muscle. This process can be repeated two more times if needed, and you will get a further stretch by the third time. At some point, you will notice that you hit your sticking point, where you cannot stretch and relax that muscle any further. You may experience pain, or the muscle may start to cramp. At this point, you should stop the stretch and then slowly bring the muscle or joint out of the stretch.

8. I also recommend that you lightly massage or hold pressure on any muscle or joint that you are working on. Again, deep, relaxed breathing should also be incorporated.

Please follow the guidelines above. They will reduce the risk of injury and at the same time improve the flexibility of your body. On my website, www.cimahealthandwellness. com, you will also find a list of stretching exercises, along with the respective muscles and joints that they are designed to stretch. These stretches stretch every major joint and every major muscle group through every possible range of motion for that joint. You start the stretches in a non-weight-bearing position first. Start lying down, and then move to sitting, then kneeling. What are you waiting for? Go to my site and download the stretches: www.cimahealthandwellness.com.

26

Your Designer Aerobic Program: Cardiovascular Conditioning

Guidelines to Follow When Creating Your Designer Aerobic Program

1. Pick an exercise you enjoy doing. I cannot stress this point enough, especially when you're starting out. Today, more than ever, your selection of aerobic exercises is vast. Possible exercises include rowing machines, elliptical machines, stair climbers, ski machines, etc. You have a lot to choose from. You can choose trendy exercise outfits or an old pair of running shorts; high-tech running shoes or an old pair of sneakers; computerized equipment or a simple road for jogging. With so many choices, there has to be something that you like.
2. Do not pick an exercise that will further traumatize an injury you now have. In other words do not start jogging if you have a nagging low back/knee/hip injury. Swimming would be a better exercise.
3. Put the necessary time aside. This is extremely important when creating your program. Remember, this is your time—not your spouse's, children's, friends', or

employer's. This is your time to develop your health, your most cherished possession. There are 168 hours in a week; you need only three to five hours of that time. That is only 2 to 3 percent of the week.

4. Develop a purpose, plan, and program before you start.

5. Stick to your program, come hell or high water. After all, you chose it.

6. Do not begin a program just to lose weight, feel better, or look better. Those goals are not well-defined; you'll be dead in the water before you start. For now, remember that exercise is not a destination but a journey through life. It does not stop because a special occasion has passed and/or you lost the weight you wanted to. It is a lifestyle change with a commitment to persevere.

7. Gain as much knowledge as you can. Remember, knowledge is the first ingredient of wisdom. It will be essential for you to read about health and exercise. Exercise physiology is an ever-expanding body of knowledge that changes daily. Sometimes keeping up is a tedious process. Today, more than ever, knowledge is a fingertip away. So, devote some time to understanding the intricacies of what you do. It will help improve your understanding and results. You will take pride in your dedication.

8. If you love the exercise you are doing, getting the results you want and having a firm understanding of how you are achieving your results will keep you going. Now, with a focus in mind and a goal to

achieve, you are ready to start your program. Let me show you how to monitor your progress, creating success with your program while reducing the risk of injury.

Monitoring and Keeping Track of Your Progress

I always say, if you are going to do something, do it right. You know you're right when you can make the changes you desire without injuries. Then, through time, your body will reach higher levels of conditioning. You'll know you are improving by measuring your performance over time. When it comes to measuring your cardiovascular performance, your pulse and respiratory rate must be determined. This is what you should measure, not how much weight you are losing. It is interesting to note that most people do cardiovascular exercise for weight loss, which is not the purpose of measuring cardiovascular performance.

As you condition your body properly, cardiovascular exercise will cause some weight to come off, but that is not the purpose of cardiovascular training. The purpose of cardiovascular training is to build up strength and stamina with your heart, lungs and circulatory tree (arteries and veins), provided you intensify your conditioning by using your pulse and respiratory rates as indicators. You must be able to take the following measurements:

1. Resting heart/pulse rate.
2. Target heart/pulse rate.
3. Resting respiratory rate.
4. Target respiratory rate.

Taking Your Resting and Target Heart Rates

When you are in a relaxed state, or arising from bed in the morning, take your resting pulse by checking it at one or two areas. The first is your radial pulse, which is located at your wrist (thumb side). The second is at the front of your neck (below and in front of the jaw), which is the carotid artery. With light fingertip pressure (using the fingertip pads), feel for a thump under your fingertips. When you can feel the thump, count the number of thumps in one minute. This is your resting heart rate. Your resting heart rate should be between fifty and eighty beats per minute. If your pulse rate is less than fifty or more than ninety and you are experiencing symptoms such as dizziness, fainting, nosebleeds, and so on, consult with your physician.

Your target heart rate is taken when you are exercising and can be measured whenever you like using the above areas. Of course, you have to stop exercising to take the measurement. People usually measure their heart rate just before they start exercising, when it should be close to the resting rate, and again when they are exerting the most effort. The purpose is to continually nudge your pulse rate higher and longer, maintaining this level for as long as you can while breathing deeply and normally (without feeling labored). You should be able to carry on a conversation. The higher and longer you can sustain your pulse rate, the better your cardiovascular condition. When creating your program for performance, please follow the subsequent principles.

If you are just starting out, set a target rate of 50 percent. To do this, take your resting pulse rate and multiply it by 50 percent. For example, if your resting pulse was eighty, divide it in half and you will get forty. Now, add the forty to your resting rate of eighty, and you have 120. This tells you that your target heart rate at 50 percent is 120 beats per minute. Continually nudge this 50 percent to 60 percent, then to 75 or 85 percent and higher. This may take anywhere from months to years.

Taking My Resting and Target Respiratory Rates

Most people neglect to check their respiratory rate, which is extremely important from a conditioning standpoint. What I mean is that your breathing has a dramatic effect on your performance. The better your breathing pattern, the more oxygen circulating in your blood, and the faster you will go. Finding and settling in on that pattern is necessary to improve your cardiovascular conditioning, since this is so crucial to performance. You determine your resting respiratory rate by counting how many times you take a breath during a minute when in a relaxed state. Then you count how many times you inhale while exerting maximum effort. This is your target respiratory rate. As I stated earlier, in order to increase your target heart rate, you have to develop excellent breathing habits. Your target heart rate depends on it. If you do not breathe properly, you will not be able to effectively elevate your oxygen capacity to its fullest and will never reach an optimum target heart range.

So, proper breathing during exercise gives you the greatest advantage. Proper breathing requires that you follow the principles set forth below:

❖ Always breathe through your nose, never your mouth. Breathing through your nose warms, filters, and moistens the air, making it more suitable for human consumption. Only during times of exertion should you exhale through your mouth.

❖ Always breathe deeply and at a steady cadence. This is important, since you want every breath to take in the maximum amount of oxygen, which disperses the maximum amount of oxygen to your body. This allows you to train at a much higher level, achieving greater results.

❖ Focus your attention on your breathing pattern, especially when performing wind sprints or when you are close to maximum effort. This takes a sound and strong mind, so hang in there.

Remember you have two goals to strive toward. The first goal is to always try to increase your target pulse and respiratory rates. The second is to always try to slow and reduce your resting pulse and respiratory rates.

Phases of Cardiovascular Training

Warm-Up Phase
This portion takes five to ten minutes as you approach your target heart rate.

Maximum-Effort Phase
This takes from ten to twenty five minutes (ten for beginners and up to twenty five minutes for athletes), saving the last five to ten minutes for maximum-effort cardio

(for example: wind sprints, which will be discussed). When achieving higher levels of conditioning, you want to intensify your routine by using methods other than time (how long you work out). Grueling sessions that last hours at a time or working out countless hours during the week can lead to burnout and poor results.

There are other ways to intensify your cardiovascular program; wind sprints are an excellent example. This procedure is not for the beginner but for the athlete or someone already in good condition. Wind sprints are performed toward the end of maximum effort, when you increase your speed to the point of labored breathing, which takes focus and perseverance. Sustain this level for as long as you can, and then slow back down to your maximum-effort level. Once you catch your breath, repeat the sprint two or three more times. Please note that wind sprints will take your target heart rate over 100 percent, so be careful.

For those just starting out, your goals are to nudge your target rate up over time. How much time? That depends on your age, condition, diet, and so on. Continually push the envelope, and reach higher target heart rates for up to twenty five minutes, and then you will be ready for wind sprints.

Cool-Down Phase

This takes five to ten minutes as you slow your pace and come to the end of your routine.

How Often Should You Perform Cardiovascular Conditioning?

Two-three aerobic workouts per week are sufficient for most people. Any more, and you are causing too much stress on the body. Remember, it is not how many times or how long you exercise; it is the intensity of your exercise sessions. Follow as many of the principles outlined above that you can, and you will achieve an optimum level of cardiovascular conditioning. The final aspect of physical conditioning comes from anaerobic (without oxygen) conditioning or progressive resistance. This type of conditioning is greatly misunderstood by most people. I hope that I can give you the fundamentals necessary to create a program suited for you.

27

Anaerobic Conditioning: Awakening the Renaissance Man/ Woman Within

Anaerobic conditioning or progressive resistance training is by far the most complex aspect of physical conditioning. It would seem that you use all brawn and no brain, but nothing could be further from the truth. Building your body into a work of art requires you to be an architect, designer, sculpture, artist, physiologist, anatomist, master nutritionist, and builder—all rolled into one. You must possess creativity and the ability to see what is not there and how to create it. Therefore, to some degree, you have to have some knowledge of anatomy (the study of structure, such as muscles and joints). In addition, you will need to learn physiology (how the body and muscles function). When you master this type of exercise, you truly are a Renaissance man or woman.

Today, more than ever, the variety of exercise equipment on the market, not to mention the jargon necessary to keep up with the latest scientific advances, is mind-blowing. I hope to guide you through this maze of misinformation and help you create a program designed specifically for you. I will give you the basics of what you need to know about exercising with progressive resistance training. I will cover the following principles of progressive resistance:

❖ The purpose of progressive resistance exercise.
❖ Terminology and rules to follow when using progressive resistance.
❖ Body monitors and sensations felt during and after exercise, which help you determine progress.
❖ How to perform each exercise properly and safely.

The Purpose of Progressive Resistance Exercise
The purpose of progressive resistance exercise is to:

❖ Increase strength.
❖ Increase muscle quality, size, and shape.
❖ Increase stamina.
❖ Increase cardiovascular ability.
❖ Increase flexibility.
❖ Improve posture.
❖ Improve muscle balance/symmetry (body shape).
❖ Improve body function to enhance your ability in any sport.
❖ Improve mind function (balances right creative brain and left analytical brain activity).
❖ Improves self-image and self-esteem.
❖ Increase sex hormone production.
❖ Increase beta endorphin release, giving you a natural high.
❖ Stimulate the immune system.

These are just a few of the purposes and benefits of anaerobic training. When using free weights and machines, you continually add more resistance (weight) to cause changes in the muscles of your body. Your muscles will adapt to the physical conditioning you give them. There is no better way to change the dimensions of your physical appearance than through progressive resistance training. Therefore, if you are tired of the shape of your body and want to make a change, this is how to do it. Stop blaming your age, pregnancies, or family traits. Dig in, shut up, and let your muscles do the talking.

Terminology You Must Know

Free Weights and Machines (the Tools of the Trade)
Free weights include dumbbells, barbells, rubber bands, and cables. Each allows you freedom of motion—hence the name free weight. Machines have a more fixed or limited motion and may not be practical for your body type. Both machines and free weights have their advantages and disadvantages and serve a purpose in your program. By using free weights and machines, you have an array of exercises to choose from for each muscle exercised. For example, there are at least ten exercises plus variations of each exercise that you could choose from for each muscle group. Surely you will find some exercises that you like.

Look at weight training the way a ballroom dancer looks at various dances. For each dance you learn, there are basic steps. In this case, there are basic exercises specific to each muscle group. In dance, once you master the basic steps, you learn or create variations of these basic steps. Once you master the steps with the variations, you become an accomplished dancer. This is also the case with weight training. You master the basic exercises first, and then you can use variations of these exercises to transform your physique. Just as people notice and compliment good dancers, they will compliment you on your physique. Just as a dancer develops grace and fluid motion, you must develop these same traits. You must practice each exercise, breaking it down into its basic component or step, which, in progressive resistance training, is called a repetition (rep for short).

Form and Technique

Form and technique are essential when lifting weight. If you watch great athletes, you will notice that they break all kinds of records by making it look easy. Their grace and beauty comes from form. Proper form is essential, because it puts the body in the starting position, which acts as a springboard to create the necessary ranges of motion in each joint required to complete the exercise. This is done with no wasted energy, creating the greatest speed, leverage, strength, and stamina, for whatever the performance dictates.

Form and technique are developed through the mind/muscle connection. To create impeccable form, you must enhance your mind/muscle connection. A person who has developed this body awareness is a champion. This mind/muscle connection requires total concentration. When you perform any sport, you must first think about what you are doing, then see it in your mind's eye, and then feel it by doing it. Eventually, through repetition, the mind/muscle connection blends into one effort, so that thinking, seeing, feeling, and reacting are done simultaneously. You catch, hit, throw, kick, and run at levels never achieved before. The more you develop this connection, the higher you transcend. Progressive resistance can create or improve this connection, since you are mentally and physically contacting each muscle or group of muscles in your body. The most exciting thing for me was to stimulate muscles that I did not know I had. In fact, before I started weight training there was not much there to feel or see. Mentally focusing on contracting and stretching muscles gave me better control in all my other physical functions.

To excel in any sport, this kind of mastery is necessary. The one way to reach that mastery is through progressive resistance, remembering that this process can take years. Ask any great athlete, and he or she will tell you that this is the true breakfast of champions. Focus and concentration, along with impeccable form, allow you to master your performance. You will excel at levels you only dreamed about before. Form and technique when lifting weight now take on more meaning, but form and technique have to be developed, repetition after repetition. Good form always starts with good posture.

Posture

I cannot stress enough the importance of your posture when performing any weight training. Posture is hard enough for most people to maintain without weights. Stand erect, head up, chest out, and with your stomach in—you know the drill. How often do you do this? You slump in your chair or car seat; you walk in a flexed posture (bent over), which continues to worsen over time until you are walking like an eighty-year-old man. My father was a posture buff and always let me know when my posture was not appropriate.

So why is posture important? Because the effects of gravity are always trying to push us into the ground, and if we do not stand erect, your spine will move out of position, causing damage to joints and nerves, leading to pain, degeneration, and body malfunction. When you were born, your body created the proper curves in your spine to maintain proper posture. Our bodies are damaged through injuries and other physical traumas over time, which create postural abnormalities. Let me explain what I mean. You are eight years old, and you fall and traumatize your spine or body. At first, there is some pain, and then you seem to be OK. Injuries to the body set up reflex patterns in your nervous system to compensate for the injury. This caused other muscles and joints to assist those in the injured areas to function as well as possible. As a child who is still growing, the problem seems to subside but when left uncorrected causes these reflex patterns to perpetuate. Your muscles are then continually traumatized by other childhood and sports injuries, occupational hazards, and aging. These injuries lead to postural distortions and the inability to maintain proper posture or gait.

I am amazed by how people walk, jog, and just plain move. Whenever I take my wife to the supermarket, I park in a way so I can observe people walking. I have seen apes walk more erectly; injured animals move better than most people. From forward head postures, uneven hips, lopsided shoulders, and head tilts it is a wonder that some people can even move. I am not here to scare you but inform you of the consequences that you will face if you live a long life, especially one that is 150 years long. When I teach patients how to stand, walk, sit, run, and exercise with proper posture, their injuries respond immediately. However, without a proper treatment regime to correct these neuromuscular reflex patterns, they will only worsen over time. Later on in this chapter I will explain proper care of the human frame. For now, here are some tips to develop perfect posture:

1. Stand tall (elongate and stretch) against a wall with your abdominals contracted (stomach in) so that your heels, buttocks, mid back, and head touch the wall. Your eyes should be level with the horizon, and your posture should feel comfortable and relaxed. Breathe deeply and slowly, and stay there for about a minute. Now walk away from the wall, maintaining this posture for as long as you can.

2. Then look in the mirror and look at the left side of your body compared to the right side. Pay careful attention to your head, and check if it is level or if it tilts to one side or is rotated. Then, look at the shoulder levels. Is one shoulder lower or longer than the other shoulder? Finally, look at your hip levels to see if they are level or rotated. Now try to stand so that your posture is erect. Try to correct any head, shoulder, or hip problem by trying

to move your body to make them look equal. Now close your eyes, and feel this new position.

Do the best you can, and over time you will see a dramatic improvement in your posture, carriage, and gait.

The Repetition

The repetition has two phases or motions: one that opposes gravity (called the positive phase) and one that flows with gravity (the negative phase). In the positive phase, the muscle you are exercising is contracting. In this phase, you exhale. Breathing is very important when performing this type of exercise. During the negative phase, the muscle is lengthening (extended). In this phase, you inhale.

To sum it up, a repetition is a range of motion that you put a joint, muscle, or a group of muscles and joints through. The repetition first causes a contraction of that muscle or muscle group, as well as approximating that joint or joints (bringing the bones of that joint or joints closer together) and is followed by a second motion that lengthens the muscle or muscle group. For example, a repetition is the movement of a weight from point A to point B, and then from point B back to point A. Please note that each phase of the repetition stimulates different aspects of that muscle and any muscles that oppose that muscle.

A common mistake I see when people exercise with weights is that they move the weight too quickly through its repetition. This will not stimulate your muscles properly and can lead to muscle and joint injury. Let me explain what I mean. During the positive phase of the rep, when people are working against gravity, they tend to move the weight faster, gaining momentum. The result is that the momentum, not the muscle, ends up moving the weight. If the weight is too heavy for you, you may recruit other muscles to help you move the weight. This is called "body English," swing, or recruitment. Using momentum instead of proper form and technique prevents the muscle from being properly stimulated, which will create muscle imbalance, weakness, and abnormal shape. Using body swing or recruitment will lead to joint damage and muscular injury.

During the negative phase of the rep, you may be inclined to use gravity to assist you. For example, if you were to perform a bicep curl, your hand would be by your side with the arm straight and the dumbbell in your hand. You would then bend the arm at the elbow while curling the weight against gravity. When the muscle is fully contracted, you would then start the negative phase of the rep, extending the arm, which is now working with gravity. If that weight is allowed to practically free fall, as I often see, then there is a good possibility of damaging joints, ligaments, tendons, and muscles. For example, a weight that is literally dropped can equate to three to four times the stress on the joints of your body, equaling hundreds of pounds of excessive force on the joint. So, never let momentum, gravity, or body swing dictate your repetition. Your repetitions should be totally under your control, not controlled by momentum or gravity. This control will give you the most out of every rep and reduce the risk of injury.

When you perform the rep, watch what your body looks like. Before starting any rep make sure your posture is perfect and that you can maintain your posture with the exercise and the weight that you are using. Watch the muscle you are working. This is why mirrors are important, so that you can see what you are doing. Remember: If you do not look good doing the exercise, your body will not look any better after the exercise is performed. If you don't like the way your body looks while performing a particular exercise, check your form. Move your arms, change your grip, use less weight, and so on, until your form looks good. By properly applying these principles, you can use progressive resistance to transform your body into a work of art. Just as a sculptor uses different hammers and chisels, you use high-, medium-, and low-rep sets with different exercises to create the body of your dreams.

Repetition Time

The time required to perform a rep properly, with mental and physical control, takes about six to ten seconds (three to five seconds for each phase with a slight pause between). Anything faster and you are wasting time and risking physical damage, especially when using heavy weight. By the way, when you slow your reps down to this pace, you will notice that you cannot use as much weight, which further reduces the risk of injury.

The Set

A set is the number of repetitions done at the same time to stimulate a muscle's shape, size, and strength. Therefore, the purpose of a set when using weights is to stimulate the muscle in order to change the shape, size, and strength of the muscle. As stated above, progressive resistance can shape and sculpt the body. Of course, this takes time, knowledge, and experience, but this is a lifelong quest. Progressive resistance can change the size of a muscle, making it smaller or larger. Let's say you have big, muscular thighs. Proper application of progressive resistance can make them smaller and leaner. Let's say you want to gain muscle in an area where your body sags, such as your buttocks, thighs, or stomach. By using a different application of progressive resistance, you add muscle mass and size. Following the principles below will give you the repetition ranges that affect muscle size, shape, and strength.

- ❖ Low-rep ranges (three to six) give you a lot of strength, a lot of size, and little shape.
- ❖ Medium-rep ranges (six to twelve) give you slightly less strength and size. However, medium reps give you much better shaping capabilities, especially when you approach the twelfth rep. The more reps you do, the less size and strength you develop.
- ❖ High-rep ranges (twelve to fifteen) are intended to tone, firm, and shape the muscle without adding size. These ranges will decrease muscle size. In fact, by using high-rep ranges, you can decrease the size of a muscle, especially if you were using a low-rep range before.

Remember, the quality of each set is only as good as the quality of each rep. If you do poor-quality reps, you will create a poor-quality set with little result. You should perform your reps slowly, always controlling the weight instead of letting the weight control you.

Another very important aspect of the set is that is does not end when you reach some arbitrary, magical number. This is a common mistake. Instead, the set should end when you cannot do another repetition using impeccable form. As you progress in your program, you will start to do multiple sets of different exercises for particular muscle groups. When you reach this level of training, which may take months, you will rely on the following body monitors to determine if you are changing the size, shape, and strength of a muscle. These body monitors are helpful when developing your mind/muscle connection.

Body Sensations (Monitors)

When you exercise with weights or any other exercise program, you have to determine if you are making progress with your program. You do not want to wait months to see if you are progressing, you need to know after every training session if you are making progress. So, what I did was determine which body monitors created the greatest results in the least amount of time. Before we address these body sensations, let me state that before you train with weights you should have at least stretched the areas you are going to train.

Please note that it is not always necessary to bash your body into the ground, as most people do when they exercise. Proper exercise is a pleasurable experience, not an agonizing hour spent torturing your body. Using all of the body monitors above can help you determine the effectiveness of a particular workout. This will lead to more effective exercise sessions that help you achieve the results you want. As you continue your exercise program, you will learn the value of instinctive training. This will take time and experience to master. After many years, I still find ways to refine my exercise program, making advances with my body.

The Burn

Around the second or third set, you will experience the burn, which is a burning sensation felt in the muscle. This is due to the metabolic waste products of muscle metabolism. As you exercise and work that muscle, the muscle goes through many chemical processes to cause muscle contraction. Since the muscle does not have much rest time during the set, these metabolites (waste products) increase in the muscle tissue, causing an irritation to your nerves and triggering a burning sensation. This is a good sign and should be nurtured. As you continue the set past the burn, the burn will continue to intensify. When you can no longer move the weight using proper form or the burn is too much, you end the set.

The Pump

As you nurture the burn, the pump will be your reward. Now the muscle that was brought to failure gets a chance to rest between the sets. Blood pours into that muscle, bringing it nourishment and removing the metabolic waste. This excess of blood circulating into that muscle firms and pumps the muscle, creating a euphoric feeling like the one experienced by runners (runner's high). The goal is to continue your sets, increasing the pump until you start to lose strength or the pump. At that point, your exercise session for that muscle is over.

A Feeling of Well-Being

When you finish your exercise session, you should be in a state of calm. A feeling of well-being is the best way to describe it. Your attitude is one of accomplishment and satisfaction in a job well done. Any emotional distress you may have been feeling seems to lessen as you can now think a little more clearly. This is all due to four factors.

The first factor is the release of beta-endorphins, which are natural chemical opiates produced by your brain. These opiates give you a natural high and a feeling of well-being. The second factor is increased oxygen capacity, leading to improved brain function. You cannot think clearly when your brain lacks oxygen. In fact, your brain is the first to suffer oxygen deprivation. Increased oxygen consumption creates a complete aeration or oxygenation of the brain tissue. This leads to higher levels of awareness and focus, causing you to think more clearly.

The third factor is emotional tension release. Have you ever noticed that emotional tension seems to tighten up a portion of or all of your body? Whether it is your neck, shoulders, or low back, there is a connection between muscle tightness and emotional tension. As a safety valve, you release the emotional overload into your muscles. In the medical profession, we call this the spillover effect. Constant bombardment of neurological impulses in the brain causes a neurological overload, spilling over impulses into surrounding nerves that feed your muscles, stimulating your muscles to contract. Through the use of progressive resistance, you can correct this neurological overload by fatiguing that muscle, discharging the neurological overload. Therefore, your body transposes mental/

emotional energy (stress) into muscular or kinetic stress or energy (muscle tension), and the exercise now discharges the kinetic energy, breaking the cycle. You feel an emotional release and a sense of well-being.

The last factor is the release of toxins. Each day, your body produces metabolic waste products that need to be removed. This is done through defecation, urination, sweating, breathing, and muscle contraction. With progressive resistance, you can stimulate toxin removal through increased sweating, breathing, and lymphatic drainage through muscular contraction. Toxins have the same effect on your mental capabilities that alcohol has. Toxins tend to dull the senses, affecting your ability to think clearly and logically, usually putting you in a negative emotional state. Intense muscular contraction can stimulate lymphatic drain up to seventeen times more than when your body is at rest.

Muscle Soreness and Stiffness/Delayed Onset Muscle Soreness (DOMS)

Within seventy-two hours muscle soreness/stiffness should come and go. This is a sure sign that your exercise caused your body to achieve a higher level of adaptation. Progressive resistance exercise is designed to stress the muscles via circulatory conditioning of the muscles you are training. As you take this muscle through the burning phase, you are in cardiovascular fatigue. As the burn increases to a point where the weight is extremely hard to lift, you are now at severe muscle and neurological failure. This is the point where you start to cause microscopic trauma to muscles, ligaments, and tendons. This trauma leads to a normal inflammatory process where the body repairs the damage you just created, which takes up to seventy-two hours to complete. This leads to achiness, soreness, and stiffness. During this time, rest, stretching, and proper nutrition are necessary for recuperation.

The purpose of exercise is not to excessively traumatize muscle and joint tissue (disc, cartilage, ligament, or tendon). If you are always stiff and achy or, worse yet, in pain, you are causing more damage than the benefit you are receiving from the exercise, and you become one of the many people who have to wear braces or supports. If this occurs, you need to visit a specialist in soft tissue injuries. These procedures will be discussed later. Therefore, when you traumatize muscle, you feel some ache or stiffness in the belly of the muscle and not in the joints. During this time, rest, stretching, and nutrition are necessary for complete recovery, which should take place within seventy-two hours. If pain, soreness, and stiffness last longer, then you caused too much injury to the muscle.

My body is becoming more physically fit as I mature. The criteria I use are the sensations described earlier. When I design my exercise sessions, I pick exercises that I love to perform, with weights, reps, and sets that allow me to achieve the body sensations in the proper balance, thus giving me the best results. If you are not experiencing any of the body monitors above, then your program will not advance, and you will stagnate.

Heavy Weight vs. Light Weight

I want to achieve my goals in the shortest period of time possible. Through the decades I have trained with very little injury following the principles above. I've adopted a philosophy that Bruce Lee, the martial artist, termed *the art of fighting without fighting*. My philosophy is *the art of lifting heavy weight without lifting heavy weight.* This seems like an oxymoron, but the philosophy is right on. In other words, your muscles do not know how much weight they are lifting—only you do. What the muscles know is how hard they are working.

Back in the 1980s and early 1990s, I had the pleasure of watching top-level professional body builders work out. To my surprise they did not lift heavy weight. Instead, they lifted weight that I felt was a lot less than they could lift based on the size of their musculature. I questioned them about this, and they told me that lifting light to moderate weight was not only beneficial from the standpoint of injury prevention but for muscle stimulation and growth. I then realized that weight training did not have to be done with large amounts of weight but with very little. In fact, the less you use, the better you are.

How could that be true when all you hear is that if you want to get bigger, stronger, or more sculpted you have to use heavier weights? There is a small amount of truth in that statement, but the reality is it's only a small amount of truth. The purpose of weight training is to cause cardiovascular stress on your circulatory system (burn, pump) and at the same time stress the muscles, causing microscopic trauma while limiting the stress placed on the joints and ligaments of the body. Heavy weight stresses the joints, and the right amount of weight stresses the circulatory system, which creates the body monitors above, such as the burn and the pump.

Another reason for using the right amount of weight as opposed to the heaviest weight is that you stimulate the mind/muscle connection. Let me explain what I mean. When the average person does a bicep exercise, she contracts about 30–40 percent of all their bicep muscle fibers; a professional body builder will contract 80–90 percent of her muscle fibers. A professional body builder has been doing these bicep exercises for decades and performing hundreds of thousands of repetitions, grounding in the perfect neurological reflex patterns to do this, just like any other professional athlete. Athletes hit/throw hundreds of thousands of balls to create their swing or throw. The average person could not hit a ball like a professional because of this fact. So, each repetition, one after another done with perfect form, intention, and attention to detail creates this phenomenon.

The final reason for using moderate weight is that when the weight is too heavy you tend to recruit other muscles in order to lift it. This leads to placing the load on other muscles rather than the intended muscle group.

The Art of Posing

One of the best ways to get your mind/muscle connection firing is to pose. I know that you may think that this is narcissistic, but the purpose is to use as many muscles as possible, creating the proper and perfect neurological reflex patterns to contract all of the muscles necessary to perform the pose.

Posing is probably the hardest thing that you can do. You are contracting all of your muscles in the upper and lower body, with perfect posture going from pose to pose.

Fifteen minutes of proper posing will cause your whole body to break into a sweat and at the same time create an aesthetic, functioning, and beautiful body.

The Use of Rollers

There are many people using rollers today to help break up abnormal reflex patterns, allowing the muscles to relax. Without going into too much detail, there a nerve endings in the belly of your muscles that work on the stretch principle. As the muscle stretches and overstretches, it gets to a dangerous magnitude, and this reflex prevents the muscle from being torn away from the bone. The nerve ending is called a muscle spindle. So if your injury occurred while you were overstretching muscle—for example, reaching for a ball in tennis or baseball—you would stimulate this reflex. When stimulated, any additional stretching will cause this reflex to contract harder. So stretching with these injuries does not work, and the use of a roller does. For more information on rollers and how to use them correctly, you can visit our website at www.cimahealthandwellness.com.

In Summation

Progressive resistance training, when done properly, will do more for your physique and physical appearance than anything else. By following the above principles, your program will be both effective and efficient. You will notice that the exercises are divided into toning and shaping (simple exercises) and size and strength (compound exercises). Simple exercises are used to sculpt the body and involve one joint, as in a bicep curl. Compound exercises, such as the bench press, use more than one joint and are used to add strength and size to the body. Therefore, besides the rep factor, simple and compound exercises also affect size, shape, and strength.

Muscles and Their Respective Exercises

I have included the most popular exercises for each muscle group. Each exercise is listed as shaping and toning (simple) or size and strength (compound). As you continue your program, try to master each of these exercises and rotate them when changing your program. This will give you many exercises to choose from and, at the same time, give you the ultimate muscle stimulation. You could add some other exercises to this program, but the exercises listed give you the foundation required to physically challenge the body from every possible angle. For more information and pictures/videos on each exercise, you can visit my website: www.cimahealthandwellness.com.

Guidelines for Weight Training

Simple explanations on how many sets, reps, and times per week you should exercise.

Repetition range:
* ❖ Ten to fifteen for women.
* ❖ Five to twelve for men.

Sets:
* ❖ Two to four sets per exercise.
* ❖ A set usually ends when you cannot do one more rep using correct form. Be sure your posture is perfect.
* ❖ No more than six to ten sets per body part.

Guidelines
- ❖ No more than two body parts (plus abs) per day.
- ❖ Train at least twice with no more than four weight training sessions per week. Each session should last between thirty and sixty minutes, including stretching and abdominal work.
- ❖ A burning sensation should be achieved in the muscle being worked by the second or third set.
- ❖ A pump (tightness in muscle and surrounding skin) should follow the burn.
- ❖ The next day or two, your muscle should ache, and soreness should be present when you touch the muscle.
- ❖ Always increase your weight on each set, but never substitute excellent form for more weight.

Guidelines for Abdominal Training
- ❖ Do two or three sets lying down and two to three sets of standing crunches daily or at least four times per week.
- ❖ Reps should be between fifteen and twenty-five per set.

Guidelines for Cardiovascular Training
- ❖ No more than three or four times per week at thirty to forty minutes.
- ❖ Take resting heart and respiratory rates.
- ❖ Take target heart and respiratory rates; do not exceed more than 80–85 percent of resting heart rate.
- ❖ Always write down time and distance, and rarely go for more time, but increase distance.

<u>Guidelines for Stretching</u>

❖ Stretch daily for twenty to thirty minutes.

❖ It may be a good idea to stretch two times a day on the days you train. Stretch once before training and then again in the evening.

28

Care of the Human Frame

So far I have discussed how to condition the human frame, making your body tough and strong to withstand the physical demands of everyday life. Now I would like to discuss how to care for the human frame. Just as a high-performance race car makes pit stops, your body requires the same type of treatment. Your life can be considered a race. Some days are like the Indy 500, others like a quick quarter mile, and others like a demolition derby. It's no wonder our physical bodies take such a beating. With the effects of gravity, temperature, light, radiation, and so on, your physical body is constantly under stress. How you sit, what you sit on, how you stand, twist, bend, lift, walk, and sleep all have dramatic effects on your frame. If this were not bad enough, consider the falls, accidents, traumas, sports injuries, and occupational hazards that we face daily. On top of this, most people are overweight, with little muscle to support the framework of the body.

{ *If the government could condemn your body, the way it condemns buildings, most people would not have a place to live.* }

In fact, over the last thirty-five years, I have seen many condemned bodies. I know I would not want to live in them. It is no wonder why Thomas A. Edison envisioned the doctor of the future as a physician who cared for the human frame. The human frame cannot be healthy without care. Let me repeat and be emphatic about this point. You cannot be healthy without caring for

> *The doctor of the future will give no medicine, but will interest his patients in care of the human frame, in diet and the cause and prevention of disease.*
> —Thomas a. Edison

your frame. Just as you cannot continually race a car without servicing it, you must continually care for and service your vehicle—your body—if you want to be healthy. So how do you care for the human frame? For the last thirty-five years, I have explored many physical treatments that care for the human frame. I have successfully treated tens of thousands of patients for physical conditions that have plagued them for years. Each treatment is discussed in detail with explanations and rationale.

How the Body Functions

In order to fix anything, you have to know how it works. The same holds true for your body. I know that most of this information was already explained, but feel that it will add to your understanding by putting it in a different perspective. When you know how your body works, you can always treat it properly. So how does the body function? Your body runs on electrical energy, biochemical electro-magnetic phenomena (BEM). The foods you eat are the raw materials necessary to produce this energy. This energy is produced and distributed to all body cells (all one hundred trillion). Your brain, spinal cord, and nervous system coordinate and control this distribution of energy to the cells. In fact, the purpose of your brain and spinal cord is to control and coordinate the function of all the systems, organs, and cells in the body. This electrical energy then powers each cell, just as the electricity in your house powers your appliances. Without power, your appliances do not work; with power, they do. Your cells are no different. With power, they can work and produce what they are supposed to produce. Affect the electrical output to a cell (like a short circuit), and the cell cannot keep up with the demands of life; it becomes damaged.

For example, if the electrical supply to a heart cell is altered, that cell cannot contract the way it should. If you have enough cells affected by this weakened nerve supply, you may suffer a heart attack. The brain and nervous system not only act as a distribution channel for this BEM, they also act as a communication channel for each cell. Your brain communicates with all cells. The cells communicate with the brain through these telephone lines called nerves. If your cell needs anything, it asks the brain. The brain interprets and creates what is needed and wanted by that cell. If the telephone lines are down, the brain cannot communicate with the cells properly. Therefore, a time lag develops in communication, and cells cannot get what they need in time to do their job, whatever it may be. It is during this time that your cells cannot keep up with the demands (remember the law of supply and demand) of the body's daily activity and can become damaged. This damage reduces the output of any chemical that the cell might produce, such as enzymes, antibodies, and hormones. This then leads to many disease processes that affect our nation today.

Your body functions through neurological energy (electrical). Anything that alters that energy affects body function. Therefore, any pressure, damage, or nerve irritation can cause serious bodily damage. Since your nervous system is so vital to your survival, it is a well-protected system.

How the Body Protects Your Nervous System

Your brain is housed in your skull, and your spinal cord is surrounded by your spinal column and pelvis, which not only protect them but also provide outlets for distribution of your nerves to all body structures. Because the spinal column, pelvis, and skull protect 90 percent of your nervous system, much care is necessary in this area of the body. This will be discussed further under "Chiropractic and Cranial Therapy." This is the framework of the body, or the human frame that Mr. Edison discussed. Everything hangs from this framework. If this framework is bent or twisted, everything else is moved out of position.

So the spinal column, pelvis, and skull protect the nervous system, and the muscles, ligaments, tendons, and cartilage (soft tissue) support the framework of the body. This is similar to the way the walls, ceilings, and floors support the framework of a building. Not only does this soft tissue support your frame but it supports your organs and glands as well. Treatment for your organs and glands will be covered under "Organ and Glandular Treatment and Therapy." It would be difficult enough to support your body if it did not move, but this is not the case. Not only does this framework support your whole body while stationary, but it also must deal with all kinds of movement. That would be an architectural nightmare to figure out. Imagine a building or bridge that could do what your body does: walking/running, bending/twisting, jumping/tumbling, etc.

Without the soft tissue support system, your spinal column, pelvis, and skull cannot effectively protect the brain and nervous system, and you develop neurological irritation, leading to body malfunction, disease, and other symptoms. It is rather obvious that your soft tissue systems will require much care if you want a functioning nervous system. This treatment will be discussed under "Soft Tissue Orthopedics." Now that you have an idea of how your body functions from a physical standpoint, let us look at the therapies noted above.

Chiropractic Care

The basic premise of chiropractic medicine is that your nervous system controls the function of your body. If nerve supply is affected, then that area of your body will malfunction. Since nerves exit the spinal column through holes called foramina, chiropractors believe that much interference occurs at the spinal level. The term that chiropractic physicians use for this interference is "vertebral subluxation." Vertebral subluxation occurs when there are vertebrae out of position that interfere with neurological transmission at that level. Falls, traumas, and accidents cause vertebral subluxations. Therefore, it is safe to assume that you, the reader, suffer from vertebral subluxation. Please note that vertebral subluxation may cause pain but not always. Vertebral subluxation may be present without symptoms. The purpose of chiropractic care is to restore vertebral position, making the spinal column more functional, while restoring proper neurological control to the body.

As a chiropractic physician for the past thirty-seven years, I have experienced many so-called miracles. I have seen results achieved through chiropractic care that defy modern-day medical philosophy. From unrelenting pain to cancer—as a physician, I have encountered them all. If the cause of your health problem is vertebral subluxation, chiropractic care is your only solution. For the reasons mentioned above, you will, can, and probably do have vertebral subluxation right now. You will need a chiropractic physician if you want to walk around at the age of 150.

Cranial Therapy (Craniopathy)

Eighty to ninety percent of your nervous system is housed in your cranium. The glands that control your endocrine system, such as the pituitary and hypothalamus, are also located in the cranium. These glands produce hormones that control your thyroid, adrenals, ovaries/testicles, kidneys, and pancreas. These glands then regulate your metabolism, digestion, assimilation, immunity, elimination, sexual characteristics, and your energy levels. They also control other organs, such as your heart, lungs, intestines, colon, bladder, etc. In the cranium, you will also find a special group of nerves called cranial nerves. These cranial nerves control sight, smell, taste, hearing, balance, and the function of every organ in the body, through a nerve called the vagus nerve.

Now that I have established a rationale for care, how do cranial problems develop? Let's start with the trauma of birth, when your head passed through the birth canal before the cranial bones were totally formed. You forgot about that experience, didn't you? Then there were the two hundred or so times between the ages of one and two when you banged your head. Let us not forget about the dental work, braces, bridges, drillings, and fillings that made your jaw and face ache. Don't forget about the time you were knocked unconscious by that fall, accident, or sports injury. Remember that fight when you were punched in the face? And remember the time when you were stressed out and grinding your teeth and suffered through those countless headaches when you felt like pounding your head against the wall? I guess by now you can see that your cranium has undergone some trauma over your lifetime. These traumas take their toll on your skull, similar to the blows that a fighter/football player receives during his boxing career. These traumas can lead to brain damage just the way they can for a professional fighter/football player. Thinking and mental focus are lost, and premature senility will be your outcome...if you make it that far.

Now that I have established the need for cranial care, what is cranial care? Your skull consists of a number of bones that are joined together like pieces of a puzzle.

Although the bones interlock (sutures), there is still motion or a slight amount of movement between the bones. This motion is created when you breathe in and out. For example, when you inhale your cranial bones move one way, and when you exhale, your cranial bones move in the opposite direction. The purpose of this movement is to help circulate blood and cerebrospinal fluid through the cranium. Cerebrospinal fluid (CSF) is produced in the brain and acts as an energizer for your nervous system. CSF works the way battery acid works in a battery. It helps stimulate and perpetuate an electrical impulse. Without battery acid, you have a dead battery. Without CSF, you have a dead nerve. Without proper cranial movement, circulation of blood and CSF are reduced. Your brain then has difficulty with neurological transmission, receiving nutrients, and removing metabolic waste. This creates neurological and endocrine distress. The purpose of cranial therapy is to restore normal movement to the cranium, the respective sutures, and cranial bones, thus restoring normal circulation of blood and CSF, which will allow the brain to regain control over your body. This requires a thorough understanding of cranial motion, anatomy, and physiology, and developing a touch that is so acute that you could feel the outline of a human hair through twenty pages of a phone book. Finding a good chiropractic physician who is also a great craniopath is rare.

Now that we have a procedure of care for the structures that protect our nervous system, let us now turn our attention to therapies that help care for the supporting structures. More specifically, let's discuss your soft-tissue structures, which include your muscles, tendons, ligaments, and cartilage.

Soft-Tissue Orthopedics

This is like finding the dings and dents in your body. You know the trauma that your muscles, ligaments, and tendons undergo to support the human frame. Falls, accidents, traumas, etc. take their toll on these supporting structures, leading to muscle/tendon and joint pains and problems. Such is the case with sprains, strains, tendonitis, bursitis, etc. This soft-tissue damage over time causes excessive wear on joints, leading to arthritis as well as disc and joint degeneration/damage. This creates joint malfunction as well as severe neurological transmission problems, since soft tissue as well as spinal segments can entrap nerves. These conditions eventually require joint replacement, canes, walkers, and wheelchairs. If you want to live for 150 years, you do not want to be disabled.

The purpose of soft-tissue orthopedics is to treat the soft tissues of the body and realign the joints so that the muscles, tendons, ligaments, and cartilage can repair and rebuild themselves properly. This makes the soft tissue more functional and provides a better support system for the frame. There are many soft-tissue procedures, such as:

❖ Neuromuscular reeducation
❖ Pressure-point therapy
❖ Acupressure
❖ Soft-tissue orthopedics

Without soft-tissue therapy, be prepared to endure a lot of pain and suffering in your life. It is even a rarer find to have a physician that can provide chiropractic, cranial, and soft-tissue orthopedic care.

Organ and Glandular Therapy

This concept at first might be confusing to you, but your organs, such as your heart, lungs, stomach, kidneys, and liver, also require physical attention. Most people do not realize the physical trauma that is exerted on their organs. Physical trauma from falls and accidents that affect your rib cage, diaphragm, or abdomen can bruise, traumatize, and cause organ adhesions (organs adhere to one another). Surgical procedures involving the abdomen and chest also can traumatize and cause adhesions. These organs include the heart, lungs, spleen, stomach, liver, kidneys, bladder, uterus, etc.

Organs can also drop, due to weak abdominal muscle support. Certain exercises, such as running, jogging, and tennis can also cause organs to drop, due to the concussive forces exerted on the body. Overeating and being overweight are other factors that cause organs to drop. This organ malposition (called ptosis) can affect circulation and lymphatic drainage of that organ, leading to nutritional deficiencies, organ toxicity, and organ malfunction. This can occur in the kidneys, bladder, uterus, and colon as well as in the organs of digestion, such as your stomach and intestines.

Procedures such as organ and glandular reflex work have dramatically helped many of these organ and glandular conditions. Organ and glandular therapies work in the following ways:

❖ Repositioning organs and glands that have dropped or have been forced out of position.

❖ Freeing up any adhesions between organs (although sometimes this may not be possible).

❖ Normalizing circulation and lymphatic drainage to that organ or gland. This helps improve nutrient supply, metabolic waste removal, and organ or glandular output.

❖ Breaking up any reflexes affecting muscles and joints

❖ Helping improve the collateral circulation between the organs and the musculoskeletal system.

In Conclusion

As you can see, these procedures can help a myriad of organ and glandular conditions. If you are extremely fortunate, your physician will also use these organ and glandular techniques.

You must incorporate these four distinct natural therapies into your lifestyle to care for the human frame and body. Without these therapies, you will not live very long in this hostile environment. If you feel that any of these procedures may benefit you, a friend, or loved one then please call my office for a complete examination: 561-627-3810. I know I am in Florida, and you may be far away. But think about it this way. If you or a loved one is suffering and nothing is helping, then you can either:

1. Continue the suffering.
2. Or come to beautiful Palm Beach Gardens Florida on a vacation, stay at a beautiful resort, and be examined and treated by caring doctors and their staff.

It's a no brainer! What are you waiting for? Start packing your bags!

Section Five:

Stress: You Cannot Live With It or Without It:
The Mental/Emotional Side of Health

29

A Success Oriented Life

If I had to choose the side of the triune that was the most important to not only your health but the success of your, life I would have to choose the mental/emotional side of the triune. I have seen people from all walks of life succumb to this side. I have seen people crushed by this side, and I have seen and read about successful people who rise above all adversity and rally to the occasion. I have seen people literally die from a broken heart, and I have seen people mend their heart through their emotions. I have seen patients come back to life even when the doctors said there was no hope because there was a loved one in the room and through the grace of God was returned to life.

Do not ever doubt the unbelievable power of thought on your health and your life. You hold the power of life and health over sickness and death. You hold the power of success over failure. You are the maker or breaker of your life.

Stop blaming others for your lack of success. Stop blaming your circumstances on the absence of success. Stop blaming your background, the color of your skin, your heritage, sex, age, or any disability you face, and start by working on the true cause of the problem you face. When you blame some outside entity, such as your boss, spouse, child, or the economy, you automatically lose control of the situation and become the effect. You literally force yourself to think that because of your child, the government, the fact that you are black, white, yellow, or blue you cannot amount to a hill of beans.

We want to stop coming from effect and come from a thinking process of cause. If I can point you to the root of all cause in your life, would you like that? Wouldn't it be wonderful to cause great things to happen in your life?

30

The Cause of All Your Problems

There is a very simple test to determine the cause of all your problems. Follow the steps below.

1. Look in the mirror.
2. The person looking back is the cause.
3. Then say out loud to the person in the mirror: "If I do not discipline myself, life will do it for me."

Whether you believe that statement or not, life will hand you your butt on a silver platter every time.

4. Now realize that you are the cause of all your problems.
5. When you can not only say it but also accept that it is all your fault, then you take control of the situation immediately.

I know that this is hard to swallow for most of us, because we have hidden behind excuses for our lack of success. We have duped ourselves into blaming everyone else but ourselves. It takes a powerfully strong person to take total responsibility for his or her thoughts and actions, especially at this moment in society, when everyone is a victim, or entitled, or is taken advantage of, or is being bullied. These are effects and not causes and are ruining your life.

At times, we all feel the impact of things that make us feel that we got the short end of the stick. Talk about being bullied—I grew up in the streets of New York where I was bullied or beaten up the moment I walked out of our apartment. That was part of life, and you either gave into the bullies—whether they wanted money or to make you feel like a piece of crap—or you hit them hard enough to give them back a good beating as well. Interestingly, as I grew up I gained respect from these individuals, and we became good friends.

Did I like being bullied or punched in the face? Not really, but it helped me to understand life a little better and realize that I would have to take punches physically or mentally sooner or later. The important thing was not how many times I was knocked down but how fast I got up, because you cannot keep a good man/woman down.

So now that you realize that if you do not come from cause and come from effect, you will use every excuse in the book to become a failure, and none of us want to fail. Right?

31

We All Possess Two Powers

We all possess two types of power:

1. Physical
2. Mental

We use our physical power to do all the things that we have to do physically to have a productive life. For example, a professional athlete must maintain high levels of physical power, such as strength, stamina, and flexibility in order to remain successful. Doctors and scientists rely more on their mental power instead of their physical power.

Which is greater? Our mental power is far greater than our physical power. I want you to realize that physical and mental power act symbiotically—as you increase one, you increase the other and have a geometric power growth. So although your mental power is greater, it can become even greater if you increase your physical power as well.

Let us explore this mental power that we all possess. There is an intelligence that runs our body and our mind. Regardless of our age, sex, color, and background, we all possess equal amounts of this intelligence. According to the Declaration of Independence, all men and women are created equal. This equality is also referenced in the Bible. So if all men are created equal, why is it that some people seem smarter and wiser than others?

The people you think are smarter than you have the same creative intelligence that you possess, but they have learned to tap into this intelligence using higher percentages than you do. It is not that you don't have it; you do not use it.

It has been said that we only use 5–10 percent, at best, of our brainpower, and the other 90–95 percent is a virtually untapped source of mental power. To tap into this reserve, we must understand what thought is and where it comes from.

As we explained in the achieving unlimited health section, life possesses an infinite intelligence capable of creating thought. This intelligence also organizes and reorganizes its body chemistry and repairs and rebuilds the physical body, using nutrients in the foods we eat. So, therefore, a living being possesses the power of thought and the inherent, or built-in, intelligence to organize and reorganize itself to perpetuate life. All that is required is to condition your body and mind chemically, physically, mentally, and emotionally.

This intelligence behind thought also runs the body. This intelligence that runs the body seems to be self-educated, and when a sperm fertilizes an egg, it does not have to go to school or be taught how to create a human being in nine months. It already possesses the intelligence to do this. Remember this intelligence runs all of your organs as well as your brain.

Just like this intelligence uses your stomach to digest food, your heart to pump blood, and your liver to detoxify the body it uses your brain to think. So the process of thought, even though carried out by the brain, is initiated by this innate, infinite, creative, spiritual intelligence and should be considered a spiritual event. So thought is a spiritual event and when used in that context can create whatever you want.

32

Thought Is Spiritual

Most people go to church to become spiritual, but in reality every time you think it is a spiritual event. This infinite creative intelligence uses your brain for the process of thought. The brain is unable to think without this infinite intelligence controlling brain function or activity, and this is why we call the process of thought spiritual. In other words, a brain is the organ that this intelligence uses to think or postulate or create. Your brain can be taught to ask questions, answer questions, add, subtract, and reason inductively and deductively. It also can store data as memories and retrieve these past thoughts and experiences so that we can learn from them in order to make better future decisions.

Two Minds in One: The Conscious and Supra-Conscious Minds

The interesting fact is that we all have two minds in one, so to speak. One is called the conscious mind, which we are all familiar with, and the other is the supra-conscious mind; some would call this the unconscious mind, which we are not very familiar with. I will now explain these different minds—how they work, the differences between each and, how you can use both together as a team to create the life of your dreams. If you can create a harmonic modulated resonance between the two minds, you will possess the greatest potential for power.

To simplify this I will use an analogy that we all know: Aladdin's lamp. When Aladdin wanted something, he rubbed the lamp, and the genie appeared and said, "Your wish is my command." Aladdin would make the wish or ask for something and the genie would make it appear.

This is how the conscious and supra-conscious minds operate. The conscious mind is Aladdin and either wishes for or asks for something. The supra-conscious mind then takes what is asked for and eventually attracts all the things necessary to achieve it.

Let me rephrase this: You will eventually receive whatever you ask for.

> "Therefore I tell you, whatever you ask for in prayer, believe that you have received it, and it will be yours."
> —Mark 11:24

I know what you are saying to yourselves right now as you read this: "Why aren't I rich? Why don't I have the love of my life or a wonderful family?"

Well, as you will soon find out, it is how you ask and why you asked for your desires that count. Our supra-conscious intelligence, which runs our body and is responsible for taking care of one hundred trillion cells, requires an organ called the brain to think with. The brain is the instrument that this supra-conscious intelligence relies on for survival in the physical universe. Because of this fact all your senses of awareness—sight, smell, sound, taste, and touch—are constantly feeding information to your conscious mind. So based on the information from your senses as noted above, you ask questions, answer questions, add, subtract, and reason inductively and deductively, etc.

The truth is that many times your senses of awareness can be misinterpreted and literally sublimated or dispersed. This is where this infinite intelligence that runs your brain can be short circuited.

As this data is being processed, it creates neuroendocrine bombardment or physiological/psychological storms within the brain and body through the myriad of neurological and endocrine connections feeding many organs/glands and other parts of the body, which create emotions, such as pain, love, fear, resentment, happiness, etc.

Once this process is complete, whatever you believe and emotionally feel is fed to the supra-conscious mind and is taken at face value, whether right or wrong. The supra-conscious mind never argues (interesting); it just does.

So let's explore how these two minds operate individually as well as symbiotically.

33

The Conscious Mind—Reasoning Will

1. The conscious mind is called this because it is fully operational when you are conscious. When you are asleep, your conscious mind is also at rest, which the conscious mind requires so it can function at high levels the next day. Without rest and proper nutrition, the conscious mind cannot function well.
2. The conscious mind is the ruler and guardian of the supra-conscious mind. It is the watchman at the gate. Whatever we tell our conscious mind, the supra-conscious mind takes at face value. If we say we are dumb, then the supra-conscious will do everything in its power to prove that you are right—that you are dumb, poor, ugly, fat, etc.
3. The conscious mind has to be educated. As we go from infancy to adulthood, we go through twelve years of education and then another four to twelve years of college and graduate school, and then we spend countless years and decades becoming an expert in our field. This is all done through conscious effort.
4. The conscious mind is analytical (left brain) and sometimes referred to as the reasoning will—we

use the conscious mind to think with, which runs our daily lives. When we are reasoning, studying, reading, writing, communicating to others, working, playing, or daydreaming we are using our conscious mind.

5. The conscious mind initiates physical activities like dancing, playing sports, or other activities that we first have to learn. Later on the supra-conscious mind takes over the thought process, and you just perform the activity with little or no thought. Ask any great players. When they are in the zone they cannot miss, because there is no thought blocking them from achieving their goal.

   We measure our conscious ability through a test known as our *intelligence quotient* (IQ). You will notice that although you may be extremely intelligent, you may not be successful in life because of other factors, which we will elaborate on as this section unfolds.

6. Our conscious mind also has the capability of motivating us to do things. It literally wills us to do what is necessary for our survival. Without a conscious mind, there is no way you can survive, and our conscious mind acts as our survival mechanism. The purpose of life is to survive. Survival is the common denominator of all living things. Every thought you have and every action you take is solely based on survival—yours or, if you are a great person, the survival of your family, group, or country. So if the common denominator is survival, then what would help increase your ability

to survive? The motivating factors that push you (your will) into doing such things (or anything) are pain and pleasure. This is what wills, motivates and drives us to survive. Pain or pleasure literally wills you to do things. If you can harness pain and pleasure and use them to your advantage, then you will have effective conscious control over your life. If, on the other hand, you do not harness pain and pleasure correctly, then you are in for the roller coaster ride of your life, with drop-offs and lows that will make you want to vomit. In today's world, we have substituted the words pain and pleasure with stress and success. We want to be motivated and driven correctly in order to succeed in life with the least amount of stress possible. At the same time, we want to harness this stress to perpetuate our success. So if the purpose of life is to survive, then you have just found the pathway to a successful lifestyle.

7. The conscious mind creates and is affected by emotions—they will make or break your conscious mind. Emotions, are neurophysiologic biochemical storms occurring in the body. The emotional state you are in will affect your nervous and endocrine systems and physiology greatly. Just look at people close to you or people you know well. Just by looking at them—can't you tell when they are happy or sad? Their facial features change—the way they move, talk, listen, and the gestures they make mimic their emotional state. I can look at my wife and know if she is excited, sad, or just plain

bored. If you look at the word emotion (e-motion), you notice the word motion, and if you look closer you see the word emote (emot-ion), which means to express oneself. So you express your emotional state by motion, which could be body movement and expression or how fast you talk and think. Just as your physical body is altered, so is your body chemistry. Your hormones, enzymes, and antibody production can go into overdrive when stressed and lead to increases in adrenalin and cortisol levels, which can over time cause excessive damage and breakdown to cells. What I am saying is that chronic negative emotional states, such as anger, fear, apathy, grief, hatred, and just being argumentative can lead to degenerative diseases, such as cancer and heart disease.

I remember when I first started my practice in Palm Beach Gardens in 1981. I was fortunate to work with a doctor who was working with cancer patients using nutrition. He asked me to work with them using my chiropractic skills, and I was very excited. After working with many patients, I found them to be angry, negative, and in poor emotional states, which I though was brought on by their cancer.

One day I spoke to the doctor about this and asked why the patients were so angry and negative. I asked if it was a result of their cancer; his answer surprised me. He said cancer hadn't caused their negative emotional states; their chronic negativity caused their cancer. That was a real eye opener.

Why are emotions necessary? First of all, let me state that all emotions are good. They all serve a purpose, and if they are used under the right circumstances, they can alter life for the better. If used improperly, they can destroy life piece by piece until you are nothing more than a shell of a person. I have seen people destroy their health, families, and lives because of their emotional states. Emotions develop or are caused from your senses, your past experiences, and how you interpreted them. They are there to warn you of impending danger. They are there as a primitive protective mechanism that enhances your survival. For example, if you were hurt by a number of past relationships you will be extremely cautious of the next one. The question comes down to how you interpret this new relationship and not what happened in the past.

Use your emotions as antennae to warn you of danger, but if you learned from these past experiences you will have a greater insight into this new relationship.

You measure your intelligence by your IQ and measure your emotional state by your emotional quotient (EQ). You can have a high IQ but a low EQ, which will cause you great stress. Have you ever seen brilliant people with tons of talent fail miserably in life? They are a dime a dozen, and you scratch you head and ask why. They are stuck in a chronic negative state, and if they are really intelligent and stuck in a negative state of anger, they are more apt to be destructive instead of constructive.

So a:

- ❖ High IQ and negative EQ spells disaster.
- ❖ Low IQ and positive EQ spells success.
- ❖ High IQ and positive EQ spells the ultimate life.

So how do we use emotions for our ultimate success? That will answered later on in this section.

34

The Supra-Conscious Intelligent Mind (Instinctive Desire)

{ Where the mind goes the world will follow. }

It is hard to believe, but unless you mentally harness and tap into the supra-conscious creative intelligence, your life will not turn out as you predicted. When I say supra-conscious intelligence, what do I mean? I am talking about the intelligence that runs your body, which is a fascinating. Although I have stated this throughout the book, I do not mind saying it again. Supra-conscious creative intelligence runs your heart, lungs, and all other bodily functions, such as digestion, assimilation, metabolism, urination, and defecation. Can you imagine if you had to do this mentally? You would be dead in ten minutes.

Just remember when you say "I" go, do, study, say, and so on, you are really referring to supra-conscious creative intelligence (SCCI). So replace the words SCCI with the word "I." So when you say "I" think, the "I" is telling the mind what to think. As stated above, the "I" tells you what you should do, say, go, etc. This now controls the conscious mind, which wills you to do whatever the "I" wants to be done. So the next time you say the word "I," be aware that you are talking about this SCCI. In the chiropractic profession, we call it innate intelligence. Religions refer to it as the spirit.

As I stated before, SCCI is part of a universal intelligence (God). It is similar to the way that a drop of salt water in the ocean has the same qualities of all the water in the ocean. Quantum physicists state the same. All matter is composed of molecules, and molecules of atoms, and atoms of subatomic particles, and these subatomic particles are literally packets of energy. Underlying this energy is an intelligence that maintains all the physical and chemical characteristics as it expands our universe. We will discuss this in more detail in a moment.

Therefore, if God/*universal intelligence* is omnipresent, powerful, and all-knowing and we can tap into that wealth of knowledge, power, and presence, then our lives will be well lived.

{ There is nothing that can stop you except you. }

{ Any question that you can ask, you
already possess the answer to.
Now that is powerful }

35

We Live in Coexisting Universes that at Times Confuse Us

Just like we have two minds in one, we also live in two coexisting universes that at times confuses us. So in order to use thought to create the universe we want, we must understand this point.

There are two universes. One is called the physical universe, and the other universe is the intelligence that created the physical universe (*God/universal intelligence*). Both are described below.

The Physical Universe (Quantum Physics or the Quantum Field)

Look around you. Everything you see, from galaxies, stars, planets, minerals, plants, the animal kingdom, and the human race is composed of molecules. Molecules are composed of atoms, and atoms are composed of subatomic particles, and these subatomic particles are tiny bits of energy. So down to the deepest level, we are all composed of this energy. The combination of these subatomic particles produce different atoms, and combinations of different atoms produce different molecules, and these molecules form different chemicals and physical structures, giving them their qualities and characteristics. So we have physical laws (science of physics) and chemical laws (science of chemistry) that help us explain the physical universe. For example, when we put exact amounts of sodium and chloride together, we form sodium chloride (salt) in exact amounts. We learn that all chemicals react in a certain way, not sometimes but all the time. In the physical universe on earth, we have gravity. It is not a sometimes law: it is an all or nothing law. You can be in Japan or New York, and if you fall from five feet off the ground, you hit the ground just as hard no matter where you are.

So we have exact laws in chemistry that explain how these chemicals are attracted to one another or repel each other. There are exact laws in physics, such as *every action has an opposite and equal reaction*, and *two objects cannot occupy the same space at the same time*. Every law works perfectly every time. As I stated above, there are fields in chemistry and physics that try to figure these laws out. My question to you is: Do you think there is an intelligence that allows our universe to exist and maintain these laws? If you said no, then tell me who is in charge. You?

The second universe. There is an underlying intelligence that all things are made from that permeates, penetrates, and fills the interspaces of the universe. Without this intelligence, the universe would be chaotic instead of a cosmos. If we are speaking in religious terms, this intelligence can be called God. Therefore if we have a piece of this all-knowing, all-powerful, and omnipresent intelligence in each of us operating as our supra-conscious creative intelligence, you can see why I speak of thought or the process of thought as a spiritual event. If you are religious, think of God as acting and dwelling within humans instead of acting upon humans from some distant location. You will feel a much stronger bond when you know God is dwelling within you 24/7. Remember, God or universal intelligence is omnipresent, omnipotent, and omniscient.

The purpose of this God, universal intelligence, the great spirit, Allah, and please forgive me if I have not mentioned your God's name, is to continue to create and expand the physical universe, which quantum physicists say is continuing to happen. This God or universal intelligence uses us to do just that through our thoughts and works. This universal intelligence lives through us and we in turn live through and because of this intelligence. So, God lives through us, creating and expanding our universe.

This intelligence wants us to have a purpose, which you will soon see is to create the greatest good for the greatest number of people. When we do not follow that golden rule and do things for selfish reasons or for personal gain, you oppose the flow of this intelligence, creating havoc, pain, and suffering in your life and the lives of others around you.

36

Knowing How to Use Which Mind

The problem we all face is that we underestimate the power of our supra-conscious mind, which is part of this universal intelligence, and use our conscious minds to control our lives instead of tapping into supra-conscious creative intelligence. How is this possible?

As stated above, our conscious mind literally communicates with this supra-conscious creative intelligence (SCCI), and this SCCI then brings the thought into reality, which we will explore further as this chapter unfolds. Just remember that the conscious mind does control what the SCCI will do.

Your conscious mind is like the watchman at the gate. Whatever you let in will affect you for good or bad, so curb your thoughts and your tongue, and your SCCI will give you all that is needed. I watch people daily tell others why they are sick, poor, miserable, or just plain fed up with life. When you excuse your poverty as a result of your upbringing, you are telling the SCCI to attract more of the same. In other words, I will never be successful because of my upbringing. I was on the driving range the other day with a friend who is the perfect example of erroneous thought patterns. He hit a beautiful shot and asked why he couldn't do that all the time. Guess what his SCCI heard? The long list of reasons he cannot hit well all the time. Had he said, "I hit a perfect shot and can do it all the time," his SCCI would compel his neurological hookups to all the muscles required to swing to hit a perfect shot each time.

I hear people complain about the economy or their spouse or their health. They are reinforcing this negativity, and their SCCI will come up with all the reasons why they cannot be happy, wealthy, or healthy. Just like the story mentioned above with Aladdin and his lamp, "Your wish is my command." This is exactly what your SCCI also says to your conscious mind: "Your wish is my command."

Make the appropriate wish or command, and the SCCI will bring it to you. Make an inappropriate wish or command, and the SCCI will also bring it to you. How does this work? As we stated above, the SCCI is part of universal intelligence and can tap into this universal intelligence bringing you, through the *law of attraction*, everything you require for success. Just like this intelligence runs your body without your conscious mind and attracts to it all that it requires to survive, it can also attract whatever you require to lead the life of your dreams.

Think about it this way: if you are married, you were first attracted to your spouse before you went out on a first date, and if the attraction was strong enough, it led to a second and third date before culminating in engagement and marriage.

The *law of attraction states*, "That which is likened to itself is drawn" Esther Hicks, which means that whatever you think about will be attracted to you. Whether it is money, business, love, success, or relationships, when you ask for these things correctly, they will be drawn to you. You will find that the things you are seeking in the physical universe will be attracted and seeking you. This can only be done if you think a certain way; when you do, life goes in a positive direction.

What I had to do (and you will too) is to break my old habits of thought and what I said to myself and to others. By the way, we all speak to ourselves, and yes, that is normal. I had to learn to think in a new way. How did I do that? I did it the way that I exercised my body for strength, stamina, aesthetics, and flexibility seven days a week. Through repetition after repetition, set after set, training session after training session, I conditioned my body and my health.

How many of you condition your mind on a daily basis? I am not talking about reading a book or the newspaper, or watching the news or earning a degree or a living. That's just conscious chatter that at best will traumatize your thought process.

I'm talking about getting up every morning and conditioning your thought process to a new way of thinking. If you do this each day, over time your mind will manifest in your life, which was once only imagined. Things that you once thought of as impossible become possible and achievable. This creates additional confidence, and you become a magnet for success.

Remember, your SCCI is always telling you, "Your wish is my command."

Take command of your life right now by rethinking your way to success.

37

Conditioning Your Conscious Mind for Success

Now that we have a better idea of how the mind works, let us spend the rest of this section on how to think in a way that cultivates our lifestyle.

Before we do this, let us look at a law called *cause and effect*. It is a very simple law that states: for every cause, there is an effect. For example: you have no money and are broke. That is the effect and not the cause. The cause is you spend too much, or you do not make enough money or worse—both. You have pain, and the doctor gives you pain medication. The pain is an effect of something and not the cause.

Hint, hint. If a problem in your life seems to follow you around like your shadow, you are probably focusing on the effect and not the cause. For example, being married three times or always being broke and unhappy.

How do I know this? When you get to the cause of any problem or situation you face, it disappears.

So follow the steps below to condition your mind.

1. Make the time to retrain your thought process.

   ❖ Give yourself at least twenty to thirty minutes a day of uninterrupted time seven days a week.

   ❖ If anything is bothering you and you have your attention on the problem, then you will have to work through the problem before you can go on. The steps below will guide you through this as well.

   ❖ Make sure that you are comfortable and in a calm and relaxed state, breathing deeply and slowly with your eyes closed if you like.

2. Be grateful for what you have. Remember, if you look at your shortcomings instead of being grateful for what you already have or possess, two things will happen. You will not be given more, and what you already have will be taken away from you. Do you see how this works? If you are ungrateful for what you now have or possess, it will be taken away. Why? If you are not grateful and complain about what you have, the SCCI hears that you are not happy with these shortcomings and will take them away from you. You might say something like, "Why do I have to suffer financially when so many others are not?" The SCCI interprets those thoughts as encouraging more suffering, and you will continue to suffer. Remember: "Your wish is my command."

If you do not like what you are getting in life, wish differently and command a new life. Start by being grateful for all that you have. Remember, most people in the world have little or no food and do not have homes. Some are attacked because of their religious or political beliefs. So start there: you have a ton of things to be grateful for. Start by speaking the affirmations below.

"I live in an attitude of gratitude."

"What I think about and thank about, I bring about."

{ I thank God that I am the ever-renewing, ever-unfolding, and ever-expanding growth, seeking expression of infinite intelligence, power, energy, and health. }

3. <u>Creating a Purpose.</u> Once you have completed the above, we now have to talk about your purpose in life. Prior to this section, I explained that this infinite intelligence lives through you to expand the universe for the better, thus creating more for more. Now that you know this, it will help you choose your purpose. Before we get into defining your purpose, let us define what a purpose is.

{ *The dimension of any life is measured in its purpose.* }

<u>Purpose.</u> This is a result or an effect that is intended or desired. In other words, your purpose will dictate the outcome or any result or effect that has taken place in your life. If you have the wrong purpose, your outcome will be a failure.

For example, most people get married for the wrong reason (purpose). That's why a large majority of marriages fail. I see most people failing in life because they either have the wrong purpose or worse: they have no purpose, which I find hard to swallow, but it is true. Ask others about their purpose, and you will hear vague answers, many of which do not make sense.

The truth is most people have no clue what their purpose is and where they are heading; they just keep on going in all directions. They have no idea, but they are running to get there like a hamster on a wheel going nowhere fast. At least the hamster is smart enough to get exercise from the wheel.

For those of you that do not have or never thought of a purpose, guess what? You do have a purpose whether you know it or not. Although you never defined a purpose to live by, you do have a purpose or what some would call an agenda, since our primary motivating force is survival. As you may recall, you survive by pain or pleasure, which will then determine your purpose for you. When you know your purpose, it enhances your survival, and you can then use pain and pleasure as tools or instruments toward your success.

Why would I want a purpose?

In that question you see the word "I." Again, that "I" represents the infinite intelligence in you, and that "I" wants and longs to *be* something, hence the term "human being." A human being then is animated by this "I" and first must *be* (have a definitive purpose), then do (carry out your purpose), and then *have* (wealth) a creative expanding life that enhances the potential of the human race, all living things, and the physical universe or quantum field.

The interesting point that I am making is you can be anything you want and will to be, because whatever you tell this "I" you want to be, the universal intelligence that is all-knowing, all-powerful, always present, the be all and end all, the alpha and omega, God, Allah, the Christ, Budda nature will weave, shape, mold, and bring into existence the being or the person you want to be. It all starts with a purpose, because that is what the "I" craves.

So now that we know what a purpose is, how do we create a purpose for our lives? In order to create a purpose that is viable, you must follow the steps below.

Step 1: Your purpose must serve others first and foremost. Your purpose is to enhance mankind, your country, and the world. Realize your purpose is not a servant to you; you are a servant to your purpose. Your purpose must serve others first and you second. It must benefit another person more than it benefits you. You must want to give without expecting anything back.

"Be the change you want to see in the world."
—Mohandas Karamchand Gandhi

The truth.

The greatest good for the greatest number of people is the best purpose you can have. Having a purpose will always identify the truth, because it is based on a solid foundation, and if you know that what you think and do is to serve as many people as possible with your own needs at a distant second, you feel more comfortable in your own skin, more confident. Having a purpose is the truth, the whole truth, and nothing but the truth. Your purpose is a clean statement about who you are, what you stand for, and what you do, and the truth shall set you free."

> { *Stand for something, or you will fall for* }
> *anything and be good for nothing.*

You will no longer feel insignificant; you will feel significant. You will no longer feel that you are going nowhere; you will feel you are going somewhere. You will no longer fear the unknown; you will embrace it.

Step 2: Your purpose must create a burning desire in you. I don't care how old you are or whether you're male/female, black/white, or whatever. If what you are doing is not exciting you, then you must either create a purpose that will make you burn with desire or look for something that will. When I say you, I mean the "I." A purpose that fills you with a burning desire will get you out of bed in the morning, excited to go to work, even if it is Saturday.

When people love what they do and take pride in their work, they are successful. I think it was Confucius who said: "if you love what you do, you will never work another day for the rest of your life."

Here's to the start of a never-ending vacation!

Step 3: You must believe and have faith in your purpose and your ability to be successful in it. Without a strong belief in your purpose and your ability to achieve it, you will not succeed. In other words, if you do not believe in your capabilities and what you are trying to achieve, you will never reach the mark. Many successful people have faced trials and tribulations that would have stopped the average person. Nelson Mandela is one name that comes to mind. Others we will never know gave their lives for this great nation. Visit Arlington National Cemetery, and you will see how many there are. However, their deep-rooted belief in themselves and what they stood for guaranteed success for this great country of ours. So create a purpose that is powerful and stirs your emotions with a burning desire.

The founders of this country strongly believed what they stood for, which was to create a democracy and religious freedom. They faced certain death and odds that were not in their favor. Although they lacked numbers, firepower, and money, they had what the British didn't— a belief and faith in who and what they were and what they stood for. They had a purpose! Imagine what it would have been like had we lost the war?

Step 4: You have more than one purpose.

Remember, you can have more than one purpose. If you are married you have a purpose for the marriage; if you have children, then that is another; if you have a profession or work for yourself or someone else, you have a purpose there; if you are involved with various organizations whether they are civic, religious, or political, you also have a purpose there. Most of these are typical purposes in one's life but if you had to list the three things people desire most, they would be:

1. *Health.* Without it, you have nothing; with it comes life, liberty, and the pursuit of happiness.
2. *Wealth.* By wealth I do not mean just money but a wealthy, prosperous life, a life that shares and serves others and brings you great joy. The more you give, the greater you receive. Ben Franklin lived by this rule: "Do good; do well." What he meant is that if you do good things, you will also do well in life.
3. *Love.* We all want to be loved and to love. Without love, life would have no meaning. Who are we but brothers, sisters, sons, daughters, husbands, wives, fathers, mothers, friends, and coworkers who require nurturing from each other? You would do anything for all of these people out of the love you have for them and they have for you. Without the law of love, which is another name for the law of attraction, your life would be a miserable existence.

Step 5: Are you ready to determine your purpose?
When you were growing up, the question everyone asked was: What do you want to be when you grow up? So I ask you now, even if you are sixty, seventy, or eighty: What do you want to be when you grow up?

Most of us already have a life, and whether we like it or not already have purposes. For example, I am married and have children and grandchildren. So I had a purpose for my marriage, a purpose for being a father, and one for being a grandfather. If I did not and left my purpose to life or chance, I would probably be divorced, and my relationship with my children would leave a lot to be desired.

So your life the way it is right now is due mostly to your purpose. Even if you do not have one, you do have something. If you do not like anything you now have in your life, you can change your purpose and do the greatest amount of good for the greatest number of people. Right before your eyes, things will start to manifest in your life for the better.

Step 6: Think about what your purpose should be right now.

Just this step alone may take you some time, but without it you will probably fail. Once you start to formulate a purpose in your mind, you must solidify it by manifesting it into the physical universe by writing it down.

Step 7: You must write it down.

You must write your purpose down on paper. Your purpose must be stated in positive terms and in the present tense, as if you have already achieved that purpose. For example, *my purpose* as a doctor:

I am the greatest doctor alive, giving quality health care to patients, as well as educating them in the field of health. Being an excellent physician, I read, write, and lecture on all aspects of health. I am compassionate, understanding, and empathetic toward my patients. I treat and educate every patient like I would a member of my own family. Above all, I do whatever it takes to improve a patient's well-being and accomplish my mission. Now *that's* a purpose!

So you must write it as if it has already happened. Use the present tense. You must state it in positive terms, for example saying that I want to lose weight is not a great purpose, since it is not in the present tense and is stated as a negative (losing weight) to the supra-conscious creative mind. You will get what you asked for: you will not lose weight. If you stated, "I am at my perfect weight, which is 135," then you have made a positive statement and will attract a positive outcome. Instead of saying, "I do not want to be poor anymore," say, "I am wealthy, and life continues to bring me abundance."

So when creating a purpose, use the following guidelines:

❖ State your purpose in positive terms.
❖ State your purpose in the present tense as if you had already achieved your purpose. By the way, the minute you wrote down your purpose, you started attracting all the things you will need to achieve your purpose.

Step 8: Giving your purpose power.

Let us look at what we have done so far. We took a thought about what we want to be and planted it, like a seed, into the ground. As we defined our purpose constructively, this seedling took root. As this seedling starts to sprout, it will require much attention to become an oak tree. What gives this little sapling the power to become a massive, powerful tree is excellent soil, temperature, sunlight, minerals, and water. The same holds true for your purpose; it will require the proper spiritual nourishment to make your purpose all-consuming and powerful. The following techniques will give your purpose power:

❖ Idealization
❖ Visualization
❖ Emotionalization
❖ Affirmation
❖ Realization
❖ Manifestation
❖ Materialization

This is probably the best explanation into how a thought in the spiritual universe eventually attracts what is wanted and brings into manifestation the object, thing, or person that was once only imagined in the mind (spiritual universe).

Idealization. When you wrote your purpose down you wrote down an ideal. This is who you are now and what you have achieved.

Visualization. Visualization is not the same as seeing, since you are visualizing something that is being created in your mind and has not manifested into the physical universe. You could call this our *imagination*, since the word contains the root *image*.

"Imagination is more important than knowledge."
—A. Einstein
"If you can dream it you can achieve it."—W. Disney
"Anybody can do anything he imagines."—H. Ford

Now look at your purpose, and visualize the ideal scene in your mind. See as much detail as you can see. You should pay the same attention to detail that an artist does. When a sculptor looks at a block of marble or a painter looks at a blank canvas, they see the beautiful picture or figure created before it is exists. They see it in their mind's eye. Ancient sculptors once looked at a block of marble and stated that it was flawed and that they could not do anything with it. Michelangelo visualized the opposite, and created from that flawed block of marble the statue of David. He saw what others could not see.

You do not have to determine how you are going to get there—just picture yourself there. If you want to be married, visualize the spouse, the number of children, their sex, and any other details you can imagine. Hold that image in your mind until it also becomes crystal clear. You must do this daily and work at making the image clearer and clearer, visualizing for longer and longer until you can see the smallest detail.

Emotionalization. What gives any thought or visualization power is the feeling behind your thought or visualization. Watch any great movie or read any great book, and it evokes a deep powerful emotion to the point that you want to participate in that movie or story. You can relate to the character and may want to be just like him or her.

That's what I am talking about. You are creating a movie called *your life,* and you are the writer, producer, and main character. Make a life that can rival any great movie or a number-one bestseller, and make it happen by evoking the emotional state necessary for your imagination to do so. Feel what it would be like to be the person you want to be. Is it wealth, health, or love? Feel the feelings as if you had already achieved the result that you are looking for.

In order for your purpose to live, it must be branded into your mind. Every fiber of your being must feel its power. By developing your purpose using the steps mentioned above, you will fuel that power. Life is a journey. Your purpose is the point at which you start your journey. Your goal may be one of the many destinations you choose from.

How to improve your emotional state:

You can improve your emotional state in a number of ways, which I use myself.

1. Find quotes that you can identify with. Whether from the Bible, your favorite author, or from famous people like Ben Franklin, Walt Disney, and Henry Ford. Read these quotes before you go through your purposes.
2. During the day listen to inspiring music; read an inspiring book; or watch an inspiring movie.
3. Exercise releases toxins and beta-endorphins besides a multitude of other things that change your emotional state quickly. All of this is found in the physical section of this book.

4. Your nutritional habits will also affect your emotional states. Learn to create the proper nutritional regime in the chemical/nutritional section of this book.
5. Proper rest and relaxation are also important. If you do not get deep sleep or enough sleep, you will be very irritable.

Continue to monitor the above and watch your emotional state become a booster rocket for your purpose.

<u>Affirmation.</u> Read your purposes daily, and continue to modify your purposes and ideal scene until it is crystal clear and stated as cleanly as possible and you can be recite it from memory. Once you feel that you are there, now come the necessary steps to bring your purposes into the physical universe. This will change your purposes into a burning desire, and this driving force will forge the new way you think.

Remember, in order to condition the human body, you must exercise three to four times per week for the rest of your life. The same holds true for conditioning the mind. If you do it occasionally, it will not work, and you will become more discouraged then you are now. Do it as a professional and not an amateur. Do it every day for at least twenty to thirty minutes. Keeping your attention on your purposes/ideals is a very difficult thing to do, but the more you do it, the easier it will become. These continued affirmations reinforce who you are and what you want to be in the supra-conscious creative mind. Remember, your supra-conscious creative mind does not rationalize;

only your conscious mind does, and because of this, your supra-conscious creative mind takes your thoughts and words at face value and brings your commands into existence. So the more you repeat who you are, the more you will reinforce who you are within the SCCI until your whole neuroendocrine axis is wired to create the new you or anything you want in life.

Realization. Realization is the creation of something imagined. The more you affirm and visualize, the more you realize that you can do and be whatever you want to do and be. It becomes more real to you and more tangible. It creates and evokes the feeling of accomplishment. "Where the mind goes, the body will follow". Realization is also enhanced greatly by action or by doing the things you want to do. This will be covered in detail when we speak about the Be + Do= Have formula. During the realization phase, you will feel that there is a strong possibility that you can achieve your purpose.

Manifestation/Materialization. Manifestation means to cause something to become real or actual. Once you have processed all of the above, what you were chasing will start to chase you. You will become a magnet and attract, through the law of attraction, all the things necessary for you to be whatever you want to be. Knowledge will appear from all over, and people, places, and things will literally appear out of nowhere to create whatever you want to create. Once you are here, you have much knowledge and wisdom about who you are, what you do, and what you have. At this point all doubt and hope are gone; you know what you know;

and this is where the impossible has become possible. For example, when I started to practice, I felt that I could help all my patients, but was I sure? Not really, but the more patients I saw and the more I acted like the doctor of the future, the stronger my belief and hope became until I knew without a doubt that patients would get well if they followed my instructions. Not maybe but definitely.

Once your achieved all of the above, you have created and cultivated a mental environment for success. Now along with your purpose, taking the right action steps is imperative. You want to work smart and not hard. Not that hard work is not necessary—it is, for I assure you that you will face tough times, but when they are over, you will be stronger, and you will rally to the occasion and create whatever you want to create. So how do we work smart and not hard? First you must promise yourself that you will live by the principles below.

Principle 1: Commitment

Commitment is defined as "a promise or pledge to your purpose." It's a promise to do something. A truly committed person knows there is no turning back. The committed person never says, "I'll try," but rather, "I'll do it." A commitment is a promise or pledge never to be broken. Breaking promises leads to emotional states of guilt, failure, anger, or apathy. On my desk, I have the following quote:

Until one is committed, there is hesitancy, the chance to draw back, always ineffectiveness. Concerning all acts of initiative and (creation), there is one elementary truth, the ignorance of which kills countless ideas and splendid plans. That the moment one definitely commits oneself, then providence moves too. All sorts of things occur to help one that would never otherwise have occurred. A whole stream of events issues from the decision, raising in one's favor all manner of unforeseen incidents and meetings and material assistance, which no man could have dreamt would have come his way.

In order to be committed, you must be responsible.

Principle 2: Responsibility

Responsibility is defined as "the ability to respond or answer for your conduct, obligations, pledges, and promises." When you are responsible, you are a trustworthy person. Responsible people never blame or accuse others or justify why they cannot do what they should do. They just do it. Responsible people realize that when they blame, excuse, or justify they lose control over their condition, and when that happens, they are doomed. In order to be responsible, you must be disciplined.

Principle 3: Discipline

Discipline means "to correct, mold, strengthen, or perfect the individual." Extremely successful people are disciplined, for they know that it takes discipline to become a better person. So, when you face adversity or failure, remember that their purpose is to correct, mold, and strengthen you toward becoming a more perfect person. Whether you are receiving discipline from someone else or are undertaking self-disciplinary action, it will perfect you over time. For you see, if you cannot discipline yourself, then you are going to be disciplined by someone else. So which do you prefer? I'd rather discipline myself. It takes all the stress out of life. In order to be disciplined, you must be persistent.

Principle 4: Persistence

Persistence is defined as "a steadfast pursuit of understanding, aim, or purpose." Have you ever noticed how easily people give up in their pursuit of happiness? When the slightest failure enters the picture, they surrender. Failure has a way of destroying persistence, so let me share a principle about failure with you. Failure is good, but our society frowns on failure instead of embracing it. From the moment we enter school, getting an A+ is great while getting an F is horrible. But success is built on failure, provided you learn from your failures. In fact, you are going to fail many times more than you will succeed. Did you know that in order to get into the Baseball Hall of Fame, you only need to get three hits every ten times you come up to bat? That's right. Even the best baseball players in the world fail seven out of every ten times at bat. Once you can master and meld the four principles above into your character, you will be ready to conquer the next step toward solving your problem, which is *action*.

38

Action

Faith without deeds is dead, according to the Bible. Even Jesus, when performing many miracles, had to do something to create the miracle. Up to this step, we have taken an immature thought and transformed it into an idea, nurtured it into an opinion, given it strength so it could become a belief, and forged it into a conviction and burning desire. Now it is time to take this highly focused thought (desire) and manifest it in this physical universe. So how do you focus your thought and create the changes you want to achieve in your life? With actions! In order for your actions to be effective (doing the right things) and efficient (doing things right), use the principles below.

Principle 1: Create a Blueprint for Success Journal.

A number of years ago, my family started to grow, and we needed a bigger house. At the time, we had property and decided to build a house. We first had to decide what we needed in terms of space. We then sat down with a designer to draw up plans (blueprints) for our house. You can't build a house without them; otherwise your toilet might wind up in the kitchen. Now, if you need a blueprint to build a house, what makes you think that you can build a future without one? That is why purposes and goals are so vital to your future. A purpose gives you a starting point, and a goal gives you direction. Just like any trip, you have to know your starting and your destination. You do not just hop into a car and drive anywhere, although this is often how people go through life and then complain when they wind up in the wrong place. Sound familiar?

This is why you require a blueprint for success. It is analogous to a road map, which helps you navigate your course and keep moving in the right direction. A wealthy and successful man once was asked to give one vital reason behind his success. Without hesitation, he stated that, to be successful, you must create a journal of things to do. Before you start every day, think about what you need to accomplish, and then write down those tasks in order of necessity or priority. As the day unfolds, cross off the things you did on your list, and never remove anything from this list without having completed it. When I first started to do this, I felt great satisfaction at the end of my day as I viewed my accomplishments. As the weeks unfolded, I noticed that many of my minor accomplishments became major accomplishments, since many little things needed to be done before I was able to reap the benefits from my big success. To say the least, I was proud of my accomplishments, and as the months, years, and decades unfolded, I noticed how far I had come, step by step, and how close I was to reaching my goals.

{ Inch by inch, it's a cinch,
said the tortoise to the hare. }

It all comes down to time. Ask any aging millionaire/ billionaire if he or she could purchase more time, what would it be worth? You noticed how precious time is when you have little left? If one views time as a commodity, like gold or silver, time takes on greater meaning. A funny thing about time is that you have a past, a present, and a future. There is not a thing you can do about the past, except dwell on it. You can think and plan for the future, but you really cannot do anything in the future, since it is not here yet. So the present time is the only time you have in which to act. Wasting your present time dwelling about the past can be devastating to your life. A blueprint for success journal not only encourages you to do things in the present time, it also helps you to plan your future. God gave us twenty-four hours in a day, and the person who plans can accomplish more by being more effective and efficient. Even if you accomplish only one thing more each day, that becomes 365 things in a year, and in 10 years, it becomes 3,650 things. Any of those 3,650 things or extra steps could change failure into success. That's how it is with life; minor things sometimes change your entire life.

{ Plan your work, and work your plan }

I once took a two-hour practice-management seminar that totally changed my life. I often wonder what my life would be like had I not attended. There are many different journal and time-management notebooks you can choose from and find on the Internet or in office-supply and department stores. Since all of us have different needs, the many different forms out there give each of us the ability to tailor our blueprint for success. So what are you waiting for? Go buy one! So how do you create a blueprint for success? By following the steps below, but first let me introduce you to the Be + Do = Have formula.

Be + Do = Have

As stated above, the "I" in each and every one of us wants to be something. In order to be someone, we must do certain things, and once they are accomplished (goals), we have some type of accomplishment. In life we are always being someone, doing something, and having something. In other words, we are always in states of being, doing, and having. If your being, doing, and having are in alignment, then life is grand. If not, life is challenging to say the least.

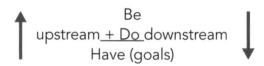

Looking at this formula, the way to go through life and work smart is by heading downstream. When you are on a boat it is very easy to travel downstream, because you use the water's current to propel the boat. On the contrary, paddling a boat upstream requires a lot more work, and the minute you stop the current pushes you backward. So you work very hard with little achievement. You seem to be going nowhere fast. Sound familiar? The truth is that most people try to paddle upstream in life and eventually fail.

For example, if I were to ask you what you needed in order to be rich, you would probably say that you need a lot of money. If this is what you think, then you are swimming upstream. If you answered, "I am already wealthy, attracting abundance wherever I go," then you are swimming downstream even if you are not wealthy at the moment. I remember Mohammad Ali, one of the greatest fighters of all time, was always stating that he was the greatest fighter that ever lived. He did not say this after he became heavyweight champion of the world, he said it to Sugar Ray Robinson, his idol and middleweight champion of the world, who at the time was considered, pound for pound, the greatest fighter that ever lived. When Ali was just an amateur, he walked over to Sugar Ray and told Sugar Ray that he (Ali) was the greatest fighter that ever lived. You could say that Ali had some set of balls for stating that, but I remind you that Ali is probably the greatest fighter that ever lived. He believed he was before he became the greatest fighter that ever lived.

> Therefore I say unto you, all things, whatsoever you
> ask when ye pray, believe that you shall receive;
> and they shall come unto you.
> —Mark 11:24

So from this formula you should see that "to be" is more important than "to do," which is more important than "to have." Now that we realize this, we must create a blueprint for success that aligns our purposes with our actions. In other words, it's nice to say you are healthy, but if you do things like binge drink, taking drugs, smoke, fight, or weigh a hundred pounds more than you should, guess what you will have? A heart attack. So the purpose of a blueprint is to give yourself some understanding of all the things you need to be, which we already decided is your purpose; what you have to do to accomplish your purpose; and the things you will have when you reach your goals and objectives. It is a road map that helps direct you toward your goals or objectives. The interesting point is that the more you plan your work and work your plan, the easier life becomes, the better you sleep, and the healthier you become.

This is simple. First look at your purposes, and then make a list next to your purposes called a *to do* list. Then list all the things you have to do in order to achieve your purpose. Next to the *to do* list, make a *to have* list, called your goals, which are literally achievements and successes resulting from your purposes. Purposes and visions rarely change, but things to do and have may change many times. These lists will never be completed and will be ever-changing for the rest of your life. The more successful you become, the greater your ability to do the impossible and to achieve things that are now possible.

Obstacles are those frightful things you see when you take your eye off of your goal.—Henry Ford

Now work your plan, and plan your work. Every day look at your *blueprint* and ask yourself what should be done in order of priority.

Remember these statements below:

1. Do whatever you can with what you have wherever you are.
2. Do not let what you cannot do interfere with what you can do.
3. Whatever you write down, do not remove until it is done, is changed or postphoned.
4. Cross off whatever is completed, and always add another thing or things to do.

So the first key to working smart is to put together a *blueprint for success.* Now you are ready for action, which is the art of doing, so follow the principles below.

Principle 2: Be Efficient and Effective. When you do things, they have to be done systematically, effectively, and efficiently.

Effective: Doing the right thing.

Efficient: Doing things right.

Most people never stop to think about this distinction. Instead of being effective and efficient, they confuse activity with accomplishment. Ever notice people (maybe even you) who never seem to have enough time to do everything they need to?

Keeping busy without accomplishing much does not follow the "work smarter not harder" rule.

We all have twenty-four hours in a day and seven days a week, but when you work efficiently and effectively you'll have a thirty-hour day and nine-day week. By the way, those extra hours and days are for rest and relaxation or fun in the sun. Plan your work, and work your plan.

Principle 3: Do It as a Professional. I remember sweeping the dust-filled basement of our apartment building with my dad when I was eight years old. I remember almost choking on the dust, and my father saw my lack of enthusiasm and said, "James whatever you do in life, do it as best as you can." From that day on, I looked at things differently. When I became a father, I instilled in my children what my father taught me. Below is an excerpt from a piece my second oldest daughter Tiffany wrote that won her first place in the Young Business Women of Tampa Florida competition.

The first question was: Who is your greatest mentor and what have they taught you? She answered:

My greatest mentor is my father. Simply stated, my father taught me the value of hard work. I can remember, as a ten-year-old girl, the thought of having to do the dishes was absolutely ridiculous! At first I protested, but eventually I relented and did the chore. The entire family was going to the beach shortly thereafter, so I was anxious to finish. My father pulled me aside and suggested that the two of us drive to the beach separately from the rest of the family. It was on that drive that I learned one of the most important lessons. My father explained his work ethic to me, and it went something like this.

He said, "Tiffany, whenever you are tasked with doing something, whether it's the dishes, the laundry, a school project, or a sporting activity, you must treat this task as if it's the most important thing at that moment in time. *Treat the task as if you are a professional in that task.*" On that day my attitude should have been that of a professional dishwasher. He said, "You must say 'I will do these dishes to the best of my ability because that is what is expected of me." He went on to explain that as I grow up and am given opportunities, I must always be aware of my capabilities, what others expect of me, and, most importantly, what I expect of myself. He would say, "If you're too big to do the small things, then you are too small to do the big things."

Taking this lesson to heart through high school, competitive gymnastics, college, my career, my marriage and my two daughters has been extremely beneficial and has no doubt contributed to the successes I have had thus far. My father gave me the tools to help me develop a sense of pride in whatever I do. Whether it is work, not-for-profit activities, cleaning, or my overall contributions to society, I know that if I do not work to the best of my ability, I will not feel satisfied with the end result. It is because of this that I feel the great need to be an advocate for childhood literacy and education programs, such as Junior Achievement and the Junior League. I believe that if we can instill these principles in others from an early age, we can not only boost others' self-esteem but this self-esteem and pride can carry over into their lives at home, at school, and eventually into their future careers. Both my mother and father have been strong mentors in my life and pushed me to be the best that I can be. I have learned so much about my strengths and that I am able to achieve whatever I conceive. My parents have taught me the values of hard work, disciplined training, and the power of positive thinking. It has been these things that have ultimately allowed me to achieve what I have, and I could not be more thankful to have them as my parents.

I just about cried when I read this, and it made me realize how proud I am of my daughter. It is not the big gifts or presents or celebrations that make life great but the simple but powerful moments that you share with your loved ones. I am proud of all my children, because they all feel the same way. Whatever you do, please do it as a professional.

A professional is always transforming knowledge into wisdom. Another key ingredient in "doing" is to know a lot about what you're doing (concepts), then be able to do whatever you are doing (experience), and then do it as a "master" who is effective and efficient creating wisdom. Therefore, wisdom about what you do not only makes you successful but adds joy to your life. How do we obtain knowledge that will lead to wisdom? First, let's start by stating that there are two categories of knowledge. One is concepts (book smarts); the other is experience (street smarts).

Concepts are simply the information that you get from reading books, taking classes or seminars, listening to or viewing CDs/DVDs, going to school, etc. Although concepts give you a lot of information, they are often others' ideas about a subject. Although these concepts help you to understand the subject matter, you must also utilize the second category of knowledge, which is experience.

Experience is actual *doing*. For example, when I went to chiropractic college, I was a dean's list student, but that in itself did not guarantee that I was going to be a successful doctor, because I lacked the experience of actually treating patients. As I treated more and more patients, my ability improved. Therefore, in order to guarantee success, you must have the proper blend of experience and concepts.

From this blend of experience and concepts comes wisdom, which is the ability to define your outcome before the fact (which saves a lot of time). With wisdom comes confidence, and with confidence, you breed success. Learning this way brings great joy, since the process of learning allows you to solve problems leading to excitement and enthusiasm. One of my greatest joys in treating my patients comes from having a difficult case and helping the patient through it. This makes me feel more powerful and confident, helping me to treat more people. As I truly gained wisdom about being a doctor, my success increased as my failures decreased, leading to more enthusiasm about what I do.

Never stop learning! People sometimes stop learning. When you stop learning, you start dying. Learning gives you knowledge to figure something out, such as how to make your life work. Over time and with perseverance, doing something over and over and over again leads to success. Each time you do something, do it better. Eventually, it becomes a masterpiece, something that you can put your signature on.

My father always told me, "James, remember this: People can take all your money and personal belongings, but they cannot touch your wisdom." With wisdom, it is easy to start over. Most people get by with what limited wisdom they have. This can lead to stagnation and rot. The thrill is gone, and work each day becomes the same old drag. This becomes boring, regardless of how much money you make.

Are you green and growing or ripe and rotting?
—Ray Kroc, founder of McDonalds

When you are bored, you are not happy, which then leads to frustration. This happens in marriages as well. People think that after they are married, they do not need to learn concepts and experience marriage. So this joyful relationship, with great love and compassion, declines, deteriorates, and rots, leading to unhappiness, divorce, and financial ruin. If you want a successful marriage, you had better become an expert. If you want to be a successful parent, spouse, or boss, you had better become an expert. It all comes down to a never-ending blend of concepts and experience, which leads to wisdom and makes you wise, successful, and enthusiastic.

Principle 4: Mastering Your Emotional State.

As you already learned, your emotional state has a dramatic effect on your thoughts, communication, actions, purposes, and goals. Your emotional state functions like a prism that can actually distort the reality of any given situation or act like a magnifying glass, focusing all its thought on a great purpose.

> *If you cannot live most of your life in positive emotional states, then you will not have to die to visit hell, because you are already there.*

It's rather obvious that it is more difficult to reason with an angry person than with a happy one. Anger, pain, fatigue, apathy, fear, hatred, bitterness, jealousy, hostility, and grief alter reality, the way mind-altering drugs alter reality. You dwell on a negative, which creates more destruction as you go. This is *the law of attraction* at its best. In negative emotional states, you never see or understand the reality of the situation or action that you are about to participate in. Facts and truth are twisted and distorted. You change pluses into negatives and negatives into pluses and focus on why you cannot rather than on why you can. It is not enough to have a purpose and goals and be educated if you live in one of these chronically negative emotional states.

I know many wealthy people who live in wealthy neighbourhoods but mentally live in slums. It's better to be poor and excited about life than to live on the "right side of the tracks" and be a miserable, mean, angry waste to society. These people are not only despised by others but are despised by themselves as well. Their lives are a living hell, no matter how much success they have achieved.

When you look at your emotional state, look at it from what I call your *typical (chronic) emotional state.*

1. Most of the time, do you feel enthusiastic, excited, happy, confident, and in love with life?

Or do you feel

2. Bored, unhappy, nervous, and fearful about life?

Or

3. Angry, jealous, depressed, in pain, or apathetic about life?

If you picked either two or three, you are functioning from an emotional state that is contra to your survival. Every thought you have is blurred by your emotional state, and your decision and actions will negatively impact your survival and the survival of others in your vicinity. Every thought that is imbued with emotions of love, success, confidence, enthusiasm, and giving, creates harmony and increases your level of survival. Rather than blurring your thoughts, they become focused and crystal clear, propelling you toward your purpose.

If you need to enhance your emotional state, the obvious question is: How do I do this? Well, what you must do is gain control over your emotional state by remembering one key fact: The only things you can control in your life are your thoughts, and the best way to change your emotional state is through repetition of great thoughts.

Conditioning your emotional state is similar to conditioning your physical body with exercise, which you must perform at least three to four times a week. You must be consistent and persistent if you want to see a physical change in your body. Conditioning the mind mentally conditions and improves your emotional state. The following principles are necessary to help improve and control your emotional state. These will take time for you to master, so be patient, consistent, and persistent. You may not live in the greatest neighbourhood, but you can live in the palace of thought. When dealing with your emotional state, remember the rules below.

Rule 1

As mentioned before, all emotional states serve a purpose, whether negative or positive. For example, there are times when a negative emotional state is a proper reaction to existing circumstances, such as grief, fear, or apathy after the death of a loved one. Conversely, an emotional reaction such as extreme anger over a minor incident may not fit the circumstances. Here's an example. Suppose your five-year-old child spills milk on the counter, and you become violent—yelling, screaming, cursing, hitting, and carrying on like an idiot. Whether the emotion is positive or negative, if it is inappropriate for the circumstances, you are having a problem with your emotional state.

Now I know that some of you reading this can justify your anger or fear about someone or something, but remember this: If you constantly live in these negative emotional states, you are only hurting yourself. You are in deep trouble and need to change. It doesn't matter how intelligent you are (IQ). If your EQ (emotional quotient) is in a state of anger, you will truly never succeed. The greatest example of this was Hitler, an angry man if there ever was one. The man was also brilliant, a genius, but because of his anger, he was evil and destructive. Being brilliant and angry just makes people more destructive. In fact, the more brilliant the person, the greater the destruction he or she can create.

So your emotional states do serve a purpose, and that purpose is necessary for you to survive. You may have learned through your experiences as a child that when you became angry, you got your way. You noted this through most experiences in your life, that when you became angry, people responded to you out of fear, and you got what you wanted. As you grew up and became a boss or spouse, you treated your family and employees the same way. *Employees need to fear me, you might think. When they do, I can control them.* This is how an innocent child can be trapped into a negative emotional state.

Any chronic emotional state that you live in is based on your survival. You trained yourself to believe that this emotional state is necessary for your survival. How do you break this chronic lock on your life? By training yourself to create a new emotional state by following the remaining rules.

Rule 2

It is your decision! Who determines, in any given situation or circumstance, what is stressful and what is not? You do! Who determines what is good or bad in any given circumstance or situation? You do! Who determines whether you are sad or happy in any given circumstance or situation? You do! Who determines whether or not you are having fun in any given circumstance or situation? You do!

So, we all agree. It is you and your decisions about whether you're happy or sad, or whether your situation is good or bad, that determine your reality. There's a famous saying, "If it is to be, it's up to me." So decide right now that it is you and only you who decide how you feel. It is not your circumstances, your job, your spouse, your color, sex, age, or whatever excuse you can use: it is you and you alone.

The following story is a further illustration. Once upon a time, there were two brothers. One was successful, and the other was a drunken failure. When the drunken failure was asked why his life was a misery, he stated, "My father was an alcoholic; what do you expect?" When the successful brother was asked what made him a success, he replied, "My father was an alcoholic; what do you expect?" Notice that the difference between failure and success was in the decision. Abraham Lincoln once said, "A man can be as happy as he makes up his mind to be." So remember: It's your choice!

> Life is 10 percent what happens to you and 90 percent how you react to what happens to you.

Rule 3

How do you condition your mind? Now you know that all emotions serve a purpose, and that it is your viewpoint that dictates your emotional state. How then can you develop more control over your emotional state, so that you live in positive emotional states most of the time and rarely, if ever, live in negative emotional states? Alternatively, when you do find yourself in a negative state, how can you get out as fast as possible? Here is a list of things you must do to condition your mind. Remember: It takes time to break old habits, so be disciplined and persistent, and you will gain much control over your emotional states.

❖ <u>Step 1: Exercise</u>. If I had to choose only one way to help improve my emotional state, it would be exercise. Exercise can help improve your emotional state seven ways, which are described below.

<u>1. Exercise increases the oxygen capacity to your brain</u>. This allows you to think more clearly. It has been shown that oxygen deficit will increase neurological fatigue, slowing your thought processes, making it difficult to think, and causing you irritability and irrational thinking.

<u>2. Exercise increases the release of beta-endorphins</u>. These are natural neurologic opiates that create the natural state of exhilaration that exercise enthusiasts enjoy. This then promotes a state of well-being.

<u>3. Exercise improves your self-image by making aesthetic changes in your physique.</u> When you are in shape, you are proud of your body and confident in its capabilities. When you are overweight and out of shape, you become

insecure about your looks, capabilities, and confidence, creating doubt, worry, fear, apathy, fatigue, and ill health.

4. Exercise gives you more energy. An interesting phenomenon about exercise is that people who exercise on a regular basis have tremendous amounts of energy on reserve, which reduces fatigue. People who are tired all the time are very irritable and cranky, because they do not have the energy to do what they have to. The energy supplied by exercise helps enhance your capabilities, creating a positive emotional change.

5. Exercise detoxifies your body. On a daily basis, your body produces metabolic waste products (toxins), which, if not removed in a timely fashion, can cause the body to become toxic and sick. This toxicity clouds your ability to think and create while leading to depression.

6. Exercise improves brain activity and function. The left hemisphere of your brain controls the right half of your body and is the analytical portion of your mind. An example of a dominant left-brain individual is a mathematician, engineer, etc. The right hemisphere of your brain controls the left half of your body and is your creative side. People with a powerful right-sided brain are usually artistic, creative, and musical types. One way to integrate your left and right hemispheres so that they can work at higher levels is with exercise. Through exercise, you create a blend and improve your analytical and creative capacity, making you a mental giant. With weight training as you exercise the left half of your body, you excite the right hemisphere, and vice versa, stimulating both sides equally, creating a mental giant that is analytical, brilliant, imaginative, and super intelligent.

<u>7. Exercise improves emotion and motion</u>. Emotion and motion cannot be separated. In fact, they are linked together: motion is linked to the physical body, and emotion is linked to the mental mind. You cannot have one without the other. For example, when someone is excited, his or her facial expression, physical appearance, and motion tells you instantly what emotional state this person is in. The same holds true for a person who is sad and apathetic. His/her face, physical appearance, and movement give him or her away. Weight training creates and improves emotional states of happiness, power, and confidence.

For every emotional state, such as anger, fear, boredom, pain, and fatigue, you have a specific neurological hookup to your musculoskeletal system. This activates particular muscles and joints to cause a particular set of fixations to these areas, creating the specific physical appearance and motion specific for that emotional state. An example would be an excited person moving quickly, or a bored, apathetic person moving slowly or not at all.

This holds true chemically as well. For example, chronic states of fear cause various hormonal releases, such as adrenaline and cortisol from your adrenal glands, which eventually weaken and damage your organs/glands and overall health. If you took a person who was in a chronic state of anger, his physical body would be locked into that position or distortion. This distortion or locked body structure would then reinforce the emotional state of anger as well as the specific chemicals released. In other words, things could be great, but because your body remains in the distorted locked position, you remain angry without knowing why. Does this ever happen to you? Through exercise, these distortions are released, giving you an emotional high.

❖ Step 2: Nutrition. Your diet has a dramatic effect on your emotional states. Oh sure, you know that alcohol, cigarettes, and drugs, both medicinal and street types, can alter your awareness, but did you know that

  ❖ chemicals, such as preservatives, additives, dyes, and coloring can have a toxic sedative or stimulative effect on your health and your emotional state?

  ❖ junk foods with high simple sugar content, such as candy, soda, and so on, can act as stimulants or depressants by altering your blood sugar levels in your brain, creating foggy, confused, tired thinking?

  ❖ low-calorie or fad diets can create an emotional roller coaster and wreak havoc with your mind, as well as your health?

  ❖ overeating, besides causing weight gain, also leads to a lethargic mind that processes information slowly and engages in "foggy" thinking?

  ❖ poor diets that lack essential vitamins and minerals can affect the central nervous system dramatically, causing emotional duress by altering the chemistry of the brain, preventing proper neurologic function, and creating emotional instability?

As you can readily see, bad diet and bad moods go together like a horse and carriage!

- ❖ <u>Step 3: Rest.</u> If the quality or quantity of your sleep is affected, your emotional state will also be affected. During sleep, your body/mind re-energizes or recharges itself. If you lack sleep or have disrupted sleep, your body cannot reenergize, which leads to mental fatigue. It has been noted in many studies that sleep deprivation or deprivation of deep sleep leads to mental irritability and depression. As you age, most people will tell you that they have a difficult time sleeping. Therefore their bodies are not regenerating but degenerating.
- ❖ Below are tips to help improve your sleep patterns:
  - ❖ Get the best mattress, head and body pillow that will support the curves in your neck, lower back and will support the pelvis. Remember one-third of your life (eight hours a day) is in bed so be comfortable.

    Finding the right mattress and pillow may require trial and error, but it will be worth it. Sleep on your back with a cervical (neck) pillow behind your neck supporting your neck and cradling your skull. A body pillow is used under your knees, or when you sleep on your side a body pillow can be used between your knees. When you find the right pillows and mattress you will sleep like a baby

❖ Regulate the amount of darkness, temperature and sound to make sleep a more pleasurable experience.

❖ Exercise helps create a state of well-being and quiets the tension in the body.

❖ Proper nutrition is important. Eating too much or too little before bed may cause insomnia or nightmares.

❖ Start stretching before bedtime, which relaxes your body.

❖ Start deep breathing exercises when going to bed. Inhale for a count of five, and exhale for a count of ten while visualizing happy thoughts. This slows your pulse and creates a more relaxed state.

❖ Try a glass of wine with dinner.

❖ Try a calcium magnesium formulation or various herbal teas or remedies that enhance sleep patterns.

❖ <u>Step 4: Smile.</u> "When you're smiling, the whole world smiles with you," according to Louis Armstrong's well-known song. As long as I can remember, people have asked me why I smile all the time. In fact, people can't get over how happy I am. My answer is, "If I stop smiling, I'll find something to be unhappy about." It is difficult to remain smiling and be unhappy at the same time. When you smile, it shows contentment and happiness with the things and people around you. Besides, smiling is contagious. How then does one go about developing contentment? This is a tough one! Try smiling; it is so easy to do and a lot of fun. Just stand in front of a mirror and smile. Remember, smiling requires fewer muscles than frowning. Follow the tips below, and I guarantee you will smile.

❖ Think of a time when you were happy and having a great time. Remember how you felt when you saw something that made you happy. By now, you're probably smiling, whether you realize it or not.

❖ Do things that make you happy. Whether it is reading a book, watching comedy, going shopping, or doing the dishes—be happy.

This is why your purpose is important, because you are choosing who and what you want to be and do, allowing you to enjoy the process. So smile; it makes you better looking! When you smile, you are attractive to others.

❖ <u>Step 5: Positive Mind Talk.</u> Have you ever noticed that when you are by yourself and in deep thought, you are talking to yourself? More specifically, you are asking yourself questions about how you plan to handle something or someone. You then answer your own question. People always say jokingly that it's all right to talk to yourself, but when you start answering yourself, you are in trouble. Nothing could be farther from the truth. When you talk to yourself, you listen and ask yourself a question. Then you search your memory banks for the answer to that question. This is normal. Asking yourself the right questions brings about the right answers, creating excellent communication within yourself. So, conversing with yourself is very natural and could be very healthy mentally, if you ask the right questions. For example, if you say, "I cannot do this or that," your supra-conscious mind comes up with all the reasons why you cannot do something, no matter how stupid they might be. You might tell yourself that you cannot do something because you're not smart enough. How's that for insulting yourself? You thought only others insulted you. Well, you are probably better at insulting yourself than ten people put together. By asking the right question, your mind then searches for positive solutions. I am going to give you a list of questions that you should ask yourself every day upon awakening. When you ask the questions seriously, think about your answers. These questions are designed to create positive emotional states by making you focus on your positive attributes, which will enhance your belief in your capabilities, creating the perfect environment or medium for success.

❖ So, after you review your quotes, affirmations, purposes, and goals, ask yourself a few of these questions. As you ask these questions of yourself, think about all those things you want to be, do, and have before you answer. You are now conversing with the supra-conscious creative mind that has the answer to any question you have. Remember, "Your wish is my command." Isn't that comforting?

- ❖ I am grateful for?
- ❖ What am I most enthusiastic about in my life?
- ❖ Why is it a beautiful day?
- ❖ Why am I successful?
- ❖ What do I feel confident about?
- ❖ What am I proudest of?
- ❖ I enjoy life because...
- ❖ I appreciate life in several ways, which include...
- ❖ Why do I love life?
- ❖ What am I committed to?
- ❖ What truly motivates me?
- ❖ What can I do today to enhance my goals?
- ❖ What can I do today to improve my marriage?
- ❖ What can I do today to improve my business?
- ❖ What can I do today to improve my health?
- ❖ What can I do today to increase financial abundance in my life?
- ❖ What would I attempt to do if I knew I could not fail?
- ❖ What could I do at work, not only to be successful, but also to make it more enjoyable?
- ❖ How could I be a more effective spouse?
- ❖ How can I be a more serving and loving father/grandfather?
- ❖ How can I better serve others?

Please add to this list whatever you like, and be patient with your answers.I want you to not only think about the answers but also emotionalize and visualize your answers.

If you follow the above principles on conditioning your emotional states, your mind will become superhuman, and you, too, will live on luxury lane, regardless of your physical address. Remember, your mind already has the answer to any question you can ask.

{ I only talk to myself when I require expert advice. }

Step 6: Success. Nothing changes your emotional state faster than success. Whenever you are successful, your confidence level increases as does your ability to succeed. Remember, success is your ability to solve problems. Stress is your inability to solve problems.

Principle 5: Dress for Success.

Back in the 1980s, a book came out entitled *Dress for Success*. I always loved to dress up, even when I was in grammar school. To dress up made me feel special. Just as words express your thoughts, the clothes you wear decorate your body. There is something special about a sharply dressed man or women. It instantly attracts attention, and people's first impressions are positive. The first thing anyone will notice is the way you dress.

"Let your presence command attention"

There is no specific way to dress, and I will not tell you what you should or should not wear, but dress the way any professional in your line of work would dress. Wearing a rapper's clothes is fantastic if you are a recording artist or aspiring to be one. But as far as a doctor walking into your room at a hospital, you would expect to see him or her dressed appropriately.

Although there is no right or wrong way to dress, make sure that you adorn your body so that it exudes confidence. Putting on the right clothes makes you feel special and enhances your emotional state. I recommend that you do the following:

1. Make sure your clothes fit perfectly and comfortably for your body style.
2. Make sure the colors that you choose are right for you and that you match them up correctly.
3. Make sure that you pick a clothing style that is right for the business you are in and makes you want to dress up.
4. If you are really creative, try to become a trendsetter and not just the typical run-of-the-mill type. Do things that will grab attention, but do not stick out like a sore thumb.
5. Over time, create a wardrobe of suits, shirts, slacks, ties, sweaters, coats, and shoes, dresses, skirts and blouses.
6. Unless you have large sums of money, there is no need to spend thousands of dollars on clothes. You can purchase clothes on sale or at retail outlet stores, the Internet, etc. Most of the time I get compliments on clothes that I spend very little on and none when I wear expensive clothes.
7. You will know how well you are doing by the number of compliments you receive from both sexes.

8. Always dress better than your best-dressed client, patient, business associate, boss, etc. and you will go far.

Principle 6: Effective Communication = Leadership = Diplomacy.

Probably your greatest challenge and stress will come from your interactions with others. We all want to be involved with relationships; after all, what would we be if it were not for relationships? Being a husband/wife, parent, son/daughter, boss/coworker, leader, or friend requires that we relate to others effectively and efficiently. All relationships are built on a solid foundation called communication. You cannot have a relationship without it.

Your thoughts are dressed in words; and words build sentences; and sentences build paragraphs; and paragraphs build chapters; and chapters create books; and books create volumes. So the longer you are in a relationship, the greater the chance of the relationship failing as a result of faulty communication.

We say one thing and do another, or we do not listen to one another when we are speaking, because we are too busy trying to get our own point across. Whenever we miscommunicate with someone, regardless of who is at fault, it tends to create mental/emotional stress during the remainder of the conversation. If there continues to be many miscommunications, it will lead to states of frustration, anger, and hostility. As these miscommunications continue, arguments erupt, and as the relationship goes on, these festering miscommunications are so charged that when you see the person you want to vomit. Relationships become so toxic and poisoned by these deep-seated miscommunications that they are now cancerous, and the relationship is no longer going to serve either one of you. Communication is the way you will create honest, sincere, and everlasting relationships.

Coming together is a beginning;
Keeping together is progress;
Working together is success.
—Henry Ford

Whether you know it or not, being an effective communicator reduces the risk of angry arguments and gets others on your side, getting them to act with you instead of against you. Any relationship—whether it is with your parents, spouse, children, coworkers, boss, employees, friends, or acquaintances—needs to be nurtured as well as understood. If I had a penny for every minute that I spent arguing or complaining about someone, I would be a multimillionaire. In fact, I would say that the greater part of any day is wasted on negative communication about events and others, whether you are talking to yourself or to others about the people you're upset with. You may even notice that just thinking about the person conjures up a number of negative emotions, such as fear, anger, resentment, jealously, and rage, to name a few. So realize right now that you need to stop ruining your life because of the way you view others, whether it is their fault or not.

Sometimes it's so easy when you won't have to deal with that person again. It gets very difficult when the person is a relative or coworker, that's when true genius is needed to handle the situation. So, let me explain to you the anatomy of a relationship and how you can effectively communicate with others to achieve your desired goals or results.

I want each of you to become a diplomat. A diplomat is by definition a person who deals tactfully with others. A diplomat gets you to do what he or she wants in the first place and makes you happy about the choice because you feel like it was your idea. In other words, wouldn't it be nice to develop relationships with others in which they love and respect you, and at the same time do what you ask because they want to? It sounds like a fairy tale, but it can come true. Imagine getting your coworkers, friends, or family members to do whatever you ask of them. Imagine them being willing to go out of their way to do it, without any arguments, fights, complaints, or justifications about why it cannot be done. Dealing effectively with people requires the proper knowledge and tools that need to be understood and mastered. When this happens, you reach diplomatic status. So how does one reach diplomatic status? By being an effective communicator, that's how. A good conversation is similar to a game of catch; instead of using a ball, we use words.

Words are thrown to someone else in the form of a question or statement, and then you wait for your conversation partner to throw back a response. So the game of catch is fun. You throw the ball to me, and I throw the ball to you—back and forth, and we have fun. Now let's say that when we play catch, I throw the ball as hard as I can at your head, and then the next time I make you run as far and as fast as you can and then throw the ball in the opposite direction. Then I throw the ball into some poison ivy and ask you to get it. Now that game of catch would not be fun, would it? Does this sound like some of the conversations you have with loved ones?

So how then does one become an effective communicator? By developing and mastering specific communication skills. It is simple to explain, but it takes commitment, perseverance, and skill on your part to get this right. In new relationships, it will be easier than with family.

Traits of an Excellent Communicator or Diplomat

1. A diplomat's purpose is to serve, share, and inspire others in any given conversation. As stated above, a diplomat realizes that a great conversation is like a game of catch. He or she asks you a question, looks into your eyes, and listens intently to what you want. A diplomat will not interrupt you until you are finished. A diplomat may even reframe what you said to make sure that what he or she heard was correct and then wait for you to acknowledge it. A diplomat will ask as many questions as he or she can to understand what you need or want. The same holds true when the other person is asking the question. When a diplomat answers a question, he or she makes sure you understand what was said.

2. A diplomat lives by the maxim: If you want to be interesting to people, be interested in them. Diplomats make others feel special, and people love them for it.

3. A diplomat always speaks the truth. When I communicate with someone, I follow this golden rule: your

actions speak so loud I cannot hear a word you are saying. In other words, I listen to what you say you are going to do and see if you do it. When a diplomat speaks, he or she speaks the truth, and your words are in perfect alignment with your actions. By the way, sloppy parenting is when you tell your children one thing and do another. Your children are not stupid, and they will call you out every time.

{ *Leaders lead by example and not by excuses.* }

4. A diplomat always acknowledges others, whether the job is well done or not, and by doing so helps bring attention to improvement. A diplomat never complains, criticizes, or condemns others for their thoughts or actions and never tells others that they are wrong.
5. A diplomat is always empathetic (understands your problems) and never sympathetic (does not accept them as his or her own).
6. A diplomat does not have to be a Rhodes Scholar, Cornell graduate, or an eloquent speaker to get a point across. A diplomat doesn't necessarily use a vocabulary with thousand-dollar words that are eight syllables long. Good communicators use easy, bite-size pieces that create agreement and understanding with others. An effective communicator may not use proper grammar, but the people who they work with love them and will do more for

them than they would for themselves. Having an excellent grasp of your language and its grammar may make you a good language teacher, but it isn't necessary to be an effective communicator. It never was and never will be!

An excellent communicator does choose his or her words wisely, the smaller the better, adding gestures, facial expressions, and tone of voice to gain agreement through respect and to determine how to serve the needs of others. An excellent communicator takes his or her thoughts and clothes them with the proper words. You see, words are the clothes of your thoughts. When used properly, especially when writing music, poetry, a novel, or film, the writer or speaker finds the proper words to instill the proper emotion. The writer or speaker has to transfer what he or she is thinking and emotionalizing at that time. When you can use language effectively, then you can communicate with anyone.

If you want people to support you, start supporting them first. Win them to your side, and you will have a team that will not let you down. You will accomplish much more when you communicate instead of argue with people. Following and mastering the characteristics of an effective communicator will give you diplomatic status, changing your stressful relationships into successful ones. After all, relationships are built on how we relate to people, and we relate to people through effective and efficient communication.

39

A Program for Conditioning the Mind

Three to four days a week, I physically condition my body. Seven days a week, I mentally condition my mind. I consider mental conditioning even more important than physical, and I'll tell you why: You have to see it, feel it, taste it, and make it a reality in the mind first before something can become a reality in the physical universe. This is what I do to condition my mind daily:

1. I am grateful for what I have and thankful every day for who I am and the people I have in my life.
2. I read inspirational quotes from famous people or from the Bible.
3. One to two times a week I go over my *be/do/have success journal* and not only review it but I visualize, emotionalize, and affirm what I want to be, do, and have.
4. I ask myself positive questions about this and what I can do today to further my purpose in the days ahead.
5. I never stop learning, through experience and concepts, about how I can be one of the top doctors in my field.

6. I put a smile on my face; I kiss my wife, kids, or grandchildren if they are around; and I leave with two thoughts in my mind:

How can I help others improve their lives? And how can I brighten their day?

It takes fifteen to thirty minutes to do this, and it will improve the quality of your life a thousand fold. Your concentration and focus will be razor-sharp, solving life's daily problems with minimum effort. You'll feel invigorated by your accomplishments, and you'll know that the day was a victory—maybe not in money or security or any other tangible item, but you'll know that you achieved something. You'll sleep a little easier knowing that your day was a job well done, and that's the essence of life.

"You earn a living by what you get.
You earn a life by what you give."
—Winston Churchill

So there it is the first step into a new dimension of life—a road traveled that will bring many years and quality to your life. Do not for a moment think that once you read this book that you know about your health. Read this book

{ *Where the mind goes,*
the body follows. }

many times, for each time you read it, you will grow and learn something new about yourself and your health. Some information will not be relevant to you at this point, but once your journey is underway many pieces of information that were once irrelevant will make sense. Remember, health is never a destination but a journey that when traveled well will lead to a healthy, successful lifestyle that you could have only imagined.

"What is now proved was once only imagined."
—William Blake

I hope you enjoyed reading this book as much as I enjoyed writing it. If you follow just 20 percent of my advice, you will not believe how your life will change. I know mine did.

May you enjoy the fruits of the spirit in abundance: love, joy, peace, patience, gentleness, kindness, goodness, self-control, and faithfulness.

When you thought things could not get any better, guess again—they already did.

One day this will be considered a masterpiece, a book written before its time. I know I already see in my mind's eye the billions of people who will live as long as they want.

As my daughter Alex says when the conversation is complete, "Peace out."

With love and admiration to all.

Peace out.

Dr. James P. Cima

About the Author

B orn in New York City on October 10, 1948, I was one of the first wave of baby boomers. Growing up in New York City was a great challenge in many ways and prepared me well for life. I mean if you were not getting into fights, you had to use your street smarts to outsmart your enemies as well as the police. This prompted me to find another way, which was to stay in school, study hard, and become something. The truth is that I always wanted to be a doctor. As long as I can remember, that was what I wanted to be. It's funny how things worked out, because years later, my wife told me she always wanted to marry a doctor.

My early years where happy growing up in a tough, lower-middle-class ethnic mix of Italians, Irish, Germans, Polish Catholics, and Jewish people.

Talk about bullying. That was all you experienced from the moment you left the safety of your apartment. From that point on, you were fair game to anyone in the neighborhood, and you either fought like there was no tomorrow, or there would be no tomorrow. So I developed a lot of street sense, knowing when to hit and when to run. I always hung around with a tough group of friends, which most people would call gangs. Whatever you call them, they were our protection, and I was part of their protection—a necessary evil.

Of course growing up in Queens in the fifties through the seventies, you were always in awe of the wise guys, the Tony Soprano types. That was intriguing to me, but these guys played for real, and this was no TV show. One mistake and you were either dead or in jail, which was not so appealing. I am not sure how my life would have ended up if it were not for two defining moments.

Turning Lemons into Lemonade

My spinal injury and poor grades changed the destiny of my life. I suffered a severe, debilitating lower-back injury in my early teens. I also had fair to mediocre grades in school. My advisor told me that I was not "college material" and recommended that I seek employment or join the armed forces during the Vietnam years or wind up in jail like some of my friends did. You could say that I was stuck between a rock and a hard place, with few if any options. I really had no talents, and I didn't come from money.

Somehow, my adviser asked me, "James, what do you like?" I told him I loved animals. He went over to this large file cabinet, searched through all the college files, pulled out one, and said, "Here is one school you might be able to get into if you pass an aptitude test."

Somehow I passed the test and instantly became college material. I was now a proud student enrolled in a state college's preveterinary program.

From that day forward I knew that I wanted to become a doctor and that I was not going to be any doctor but a *doctor's doctor*. I studied as hard as I could and raised my grades enough to get into Cornell University's preveterinary program. I graduated in the top 25 percent of my class. Not bad for not being college material.

A Slight Shift in Direction

During my early teen years, I developed severe back pain, which was thought to be congenital. I was born with a bad back, and because it was congenital there was no way out. As I entered college, my back pain became debilitating to the point that something had to be done. My doctor did not want me to undergo surgery and suggested I tough it out, which I did, but you always heard stories about once you have a bad back you will always have a bad back. This was not fun to hear when you're eighteen, but it was true.

One day it really hit home while I was lying on the floor of my girlfriend's living room in severe pain when her father's friend asked me what was wrong. I told him my back was killing me, and he said don't worry, "It is going to get worse with age," as he stepped over me and walked out the front door.

Although it seemed cruel, it hit me like a ton of bricks. I knew he was right and that it was only going to get worse if I didn't correct the problem, but how? Had it not been for that epiphany, I probably would never have chosen the path I did. I decided to find out about back pain and was accidentally introduced to the field of chiropractic. I went to a doctor of chiropractic who helped me with my back problem. As I learned about the profession, I realized that they were able to treat many other health problems besides back pain. Well that just seemed to be the icing on the cake, because if I could just help people with low back pain, that in itself would have been a rewarding experience. That was it. I applied to what is now known as New York Chiropractic College, received my degree in 1976, and was off and running.

As I was in my last year of school, I saw a quote from Thomas Edison about the doctor of the future: "The doctor of the future will give no medication but will interest his patients in diet, care of the human frame, and the cause and prevention of disease." Although the definition was near perfect, there was no how-to manual that explained how the doctor was going to treat his patients.

From that day forward I was hooked, and I wanted to become the doctor of the future. I devoted my life to health and wellness, and forty years later I have created a health and wellness program that lives up to Mr. Edison's vision of the doctor of the future.

In 1980, I left New York City with my new bride Gloria and moved to beautiful Palm Beach, Florida. My wife and I started my practice in 1981 and raised a family of four—Natalie, Tiffany, James, and Alexandra, two of which are chiropractic physicians and now practice with me.

We have four grandchildren with one on the way, and we hope to add a third generation to our practice. Our commitment is to offer the best health care available, which we always strive to achieve. Whether it is through education, treatment, or recommendations, our goal is to *improve the health of this great nation, one patient at a time.*

Please enjoy this book. I wrote it for you, your family, and your loved ones.

Sincerely, Dr. James Cima

Quotes by Dr. Cima

1. If you don't take the time to take care of your health, you will have to take the time to take care of your sickness and disease!

2. Symptoms are the end result of a disease process, not the beginning.

3. Learn the secrets of metabolic stimulation that can transform your body, mind, health, and life.

4. To improve your anabolic phase, you must have:
   Proper mental/emotional and physical stimulation
   Proper mental/emotional and physical rest
   Proper nutrition to repair and rebuild the body

5. Your survival potential is proportionate to your health.

6. Healthy people do not die from sickness and disease; sick people do.

7. Feeling or looking good does not mean that you are healthy. And experiencing symptoms does not mean that you are sick.

8. Health: A condition of wholeness in which the body/mind functions at peak performance chemically, physically, and mentally emotionally as a triune in perfect harmony.

9. Let us prolong the regeneration of youth rather than perpetuate the degeneration of cancer and heart disease.

10. If you do not take care of your body, where else are you going to live?

11. Just like your car, if you want to speed up your metabolism, you give your body more of the right fuel and not less of the wrong fuel.

12. Exercise does not consume time; it manufactures time.

13. Worth more than riches and fine gold, your body and health are things of beauty, gifts from God that money cannot buy.

14. If the government could condemn your body, the way it condemns buildings, most people would not have a place to live.

15. Where the mind goes the world will follow.

16. There is nothing that can stop you except you.

17. Any question that you can ask, you already possess the answer to. Now that is powerful.

18. The dimension of any life is measured in its purpose.

19. I thank God that I am the ever-renewing, ever-unfolding, and ever-expanding growth, seeking expression of infinite intelligence, power, energy, and health.

20. Stand for something, or you will fall for anything and be good for nothing.

21. Inch by inch, it's a cinch, said the tortoise to the hare.

22. Plan your work, and work your plan.

23. If you cannot live most of your life in positive emotional states, then you will not have to die to visit hell, because you are already there.

24. Life is 10 percent what happens to you and 90 percent how you react to what happens to you.

25. I only talk to myself when I require expert advice.

26. Leaders lead by example and not by excuses.

27. Where the mind goes, the body follows.

Made in the USA
Columbia, SC
20 August 2019